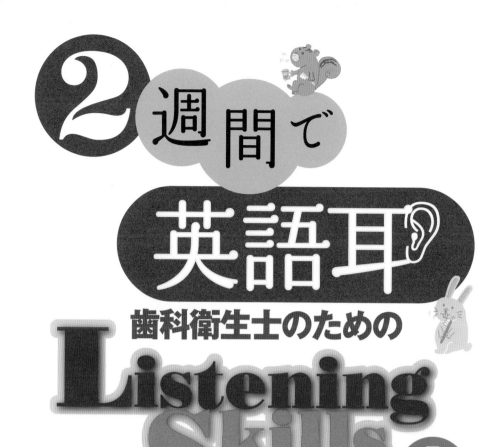

2週間で 英語耳

歯科衛生士のための

Listening Skills

音声DL付

C.S.Langham
田嶋倫雄
著

医歯薬出版株式会社

This book is originally published in Japanese
under the title of :

2 SHUKAN DE EIGOMIMI
SHIKA EISEISHI NO TAME NO RISUNINGU SUKIRU
(A two-week program in English Listening Skills for Dental Hygienists)

C. S. Langham
   Professor at Nihon University School of Dentistry
TAJIMA, MICHIO
   Associate Professor at Nihon University School of Dentistry

© 2024 1st ed.

ISHIYAKU PUBLISHERS, INC.
   7-10, Honkomagome 1 chome, Bunkyo-ku,
   Tokyo 113-8612, Japan

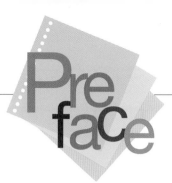

Preface

F or several years, I taught English to students at the dental hygienist training school attached to Nihon University School of Dentistry. Graduates of the program told me they sometimes had non-Japanese patients and needed to use English in order to explain treatment. As Japan becomes more and more international, the need for dental hygienists who can speak English will increase. I believe that to be able to communicate in English you need good listening skills. In this book, there are over 50 listening exercises based on situations in dental clinics between patients and dental hygienists. There are also model conversations that will help you to develop your speaking skills. At the end of each unit, there is a list of target vocabulary which contains technical words you will need to remember and use. I hope this book will help to improve your listening skills, and also give you the confidence to communicate in English with non-Japanese patients.

Clive Langham
Nihon University School of Dentistry
March 1st, 2008

音声データのダウンロードと
ご利用について

・本書中の 🔽01 の番号は音声データのトラックナンバーを示しています.

・音声データは下記の URL または QR コードから無料でダウンロードすることができます.

    https://www.ishiyaku.co.jp/ebooks/423270/

<注意事項>

・再生には MP3 形式の音声データを再生できる環境が必要です.

・お客様がご負担になる通信料金について十分にご理解のうえご利用をお願いします.

・音声データを無断で複製・公に上映・公衆送信（送信可能化を含む）・翻訳・翻案することは法律により禁止されています.

<お問合せ先>

    https://www.ishiyaku.co.jp/ebooks/inquiry/

本書の特徴

本書は，おもに歯科衛生士が患者さんと英語で受け答えをする
という状況を想定してつくられています．
学習者には，歯科衛生士を目指している学生や
臨床の現場で活躍している歯科衛生士のほか，
歯科医師や受付など幅広く想定しており，
リスニングとスピーキングを効果的に学べる教材となっています．

本書のおもな特徴は以下のとおりです．

① 各ユニットは見開き完結の2ページ構成となっており，容易に学習パターンをつくり上げることができます．各ユニットは20分程度で学習できるため，授業での副教材のほか，通学・通勤中などでの自己学習にも最適です．

② 最新の英語教育法を基盤にしており，学習者が能動的に学べるようにつくられています．レベルは初級者から中級者向けで，段階的にレベルが上がるようにしてあります．

③ 学習記憶に残りやすいように，モデル会話やリスニング問題を簡潔・明瞭にしてあります．また，スピーキングについては定型表現に重点を置いています．

④ 各ユニットの重要単語を絞り込み，利用価値の高い単語に集中させています．また，辞書を引く時間を節約するため，各ユニットには「Mini Dictionary」を用意しています．

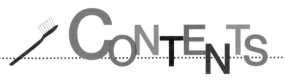

CONTENTS

歯科衛生士のための Listening Skills

以下のように学習すると効果的です.

1. 各ユニットのタイトル

　タイトルをみてどんな場面設定かを想像し, どんな会話を聴くのかを予想する (タイトルは何を意味しているのか? そのユニットを学ぶと患者さんとどんな会話をできるようになるのか? など).

2. リスニング

① 問題文を読む.
② 音声を2〜3回聴く. 最初は本書をみないで聴き, 次に問題内容を眺めながら聴く. 会話全体を捉え, 必要な情報収集を行うことを目的とする. つまり, 英文そのものではなく, 内容理解に集中する.
③ 答えを確認する. 授業で使用するときは, よく聴き取れない箇所を教員がゆっくり読み上げるのもよい.
④ 重要なセリフに注目する.
⑤ もう一度音声を聴き, 問題を解く. 時間の許すかぎり繰り返すとよい.

3. スピーキング

① 会話を読む (授業では学生どうしでペアになるとよい). このときは, 内容だけでなく英文にも目を向ける.
② 重要なセンテンスに注目する.
③ Target sentences を確認する (授業では, 宿題やテストにも利用できる). 何を伝えようとしているのかを意識する.
④ Target vocabulary に取り組む.
⑤ Mini Dictionary の単語を覚える.

Have you visited us before?

Listening 1 01

The DH is talking to a patient on the phone. Is it a new patient or a registered patient? Listen and put a check in the correct box.

	New Patient	Registered Patient
1.	☐	☐
2.	☐	☐
3.	☐	☐
4.	☐	☐
5.	☐	☐

Listening 2 02

You will hear 6 questions the DH asks a patient. Listen and complete the blanks. Then, listen to the patient's answers A~F and match them with the questions. The first one A is done for you.

1. _____ _____ _____ us before? ( )
2. _____ _____ _____ your name, please? ( )
3. _____ _____ _____ that, please? (A)
4. _____ _____ _____ come in? ( )
5. _____ _____ _____ or Wednesday
   next week at about 5:30? ( )
6. _____ _____ _____ Japanese health insurance? ( )

Listening 3 03

Listen to 6 words. Are they singular or plural? Write S for singular or P for plural in the brackets, then write the word. The first one is done for you.

1. (S) __recall card__   4. ( ) _____
2. ( ) _____   5. ( ) _____
3. ( ) _____   6. ( ) _____

Speaking 1 (DH : Dental Hygienist, PT : Patient)

DH : Good morning. Azuma Dental Clinic. How may I help you?
PT : I'd like to make an appointment.
DH : Have you visited us before?
PT : No, this is my first time.
DH : Okay. So, you need to register. First, let me take some details. Could I have your name, please?
PT : It's Jones. Bill Jones.
DH : Could you spell that, please?
PT : Sure. It's J-O-N-E-S
DH : Thank you, Mr. Jones. When can you come in?
PT : How about Wednesday or Thursday next week?

Speaking 2

Target sentences: Getting information
1. Have you visited us before?
2. You need to register.
3. First, let me take some details.
4. Could I have your name, please?
5. Could you spell that, please?
6. Do you have Japanese health insurance?
7. When can you come in?
8. Okay, Mr. Jenkins. Your appointment is for Thursday at 10:30 with DH Watanabe.

Target vocabulary 04

Listen and number the words you hear from 1~7.
(　) appointment　(　) details　(　) register　(　) toothache
(　) recall card　(　) teeth　(　) cleaned

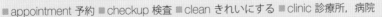

Mini Dictionary

■appointment 予約 ■checkup 検査 ■clean きれいにする ■clinic 診療所，病院
■dental hygienist (DH) 歯科衛生士 ■dentist 歯科医師 ■details 詳細
■Japanese health insurance 日本の健康保険 ■new patient 初診患者 ■patient (PT) 患者
■recall card 定期検診のハガキ ■register 登録 ■registered patient 再診患者
■teeth 歯（複数形）

Taking a patient's name, address, telephone number Filling out a registration card

Listening 1 ⬇05

Listen and write down the patient's family name.
1. Bill _____
2. Peter _____
3. James _____
4. Dave _____
5. Sarah _____

Listening 2 ⬇06

Listen and circle the correct family name.
1.   Nebara / Nevara
2.   Williams / William
3.   Sikorski / Shikorski
4.   Waldhof / Waldhoff
5.   Right / Wright

Listening 3 ⬇07

The DH is helping a patient to fill out a registration card. Listen and complete the card with the patient's details.

Name	First: John Family: _____
Sex	Male / Female
Age	_____
Address	Minato City, Higashi_____
Telephone No.	080-340 __ __ - __ __ __ __

Speaking 1

DH : Could I have your name, please?
PT : It's Jim Sikorski.
DH : Could you spell that, please?
PT : Sure. It's S-I-K-O-R-S-K-I. And my first name is Jim.
DH : How old are you, Mr. Sikorski?
PT : 39.
DH : And what's your address?
PT : It's Sakura New Town, Nishi 2-5-206.
DH : Okay. And what's your telephone number?

Speaking 2

Target sentences: Checking a patient's name, address and telephone number

Name	What's your name?
	Could I have your name, please?
	What's your family name?
Spelling	Could you spell that, please?
	Would you mind spelling that, please?
Age	How old are you?
Address	What's your address?
Telephone No.	What's your telephone number?

Target vocabulary 08

Listen to the Japanese words and write down the English words.

1. _____   2. _____   3. _____
4. _____   5. _____   6. _____

Mini Dictionary

■ address 住所 ■ family name 苗字 ■ first name 名前 ■ fill out 記入する
■ registration card 診療申込書 ■ telephone number 電話番号

3 Making appointments: Days, dates, times

Listening 1 09

Listen to conversations 1~5 between the DH and patients. Complete the grid below.

	NAME	DAY	DATE	TIME
1	Mr. Williams		3/20	
2	Mr. Jones			3pm
3	Ms. Chang	Tuesday		
4	Ms. Clinton	Friday		
5	Mr. Fernandez		4/10	

Listening 2 10

Listen and circle the correct date.
1. May 13th ∕ May 30th
2. June 15th ∕ July 15th
3. May 6th ∕ May 16th
4. October 9th ∕ October 19th
5. December 4th ∕ December 14th

Listening 3 11

Listen and circle the correct time.
1. 3:30 ∕ 3:15
2. 8:00 ∕ 12:00
3. 9:15 ∕ 9:50
4. 8:15 ∕ 8:45
5. 2:20 ∕ 3:20

Speaking 1

DH : Let's fix your next appointment. When is convenient for you?
PT : I'm free on Wednesday next week. The evening is the best time.
DH : Okay, let me check that. Yes, Wednesday, March the 20th is okay. What time would suit you?
PT : Around 7pm.
DH : How about 7:30?
PT : Yes, that's fine.
DH : So, that's Wednesday, March the 20th at 7:30pm.

Speaking 2

Target sentences: Appointments and times

Arranging an appointment	Suggesting a time	Confirming a time
1. When is convenient?	1. How about 9pm?	So, that's Wednesday, March the 20th at 7:30.
2. When can you come in?	2. Is 1pm good for you?	
3. What time would suit you?		
4. What time is good for you?		

Target vocabulary 12

Listen to the Japanese words 1~8 and match them with the English words. Write the number in the brackets.

( ) braces
( ) dental hygienist
( ) brush properly
( ) orthodontic treatment
( ) molars
( ) crown
( ) oral hygiene
( ) restoration

Mini Dictionary

■appointment 予約 ■braces 歯列矯正装置 ■brush 磨く ■check 調べる，検査する
■convenient 都合がよい ■crown クラウン ■decay 齲蝕（むし歯） ■molar 大臼歯
■oral hygiene 口腔衛生 ■orthodontic treatment 歯科矯正治療 ■restoration 修復

Special Listening

Listening to Dental Topics 1

This is a page from a student's notebook. Listen and complete the missing information.

⬇13

Dental Data from the UK

1. Oral Health Problems

① About (　) million people visit their dentist with toothache every year.

② About (　) % of adults have (　) or more fillings.

2. Oral Health Routine

① (　) in 5 people brush their teeth less than (　　　) a day.

② Most adults only change their toothbrush (　　　) a year.

③ (　) % of people use an electric toothbrush.

263-00993

Crossword Puzzle 1

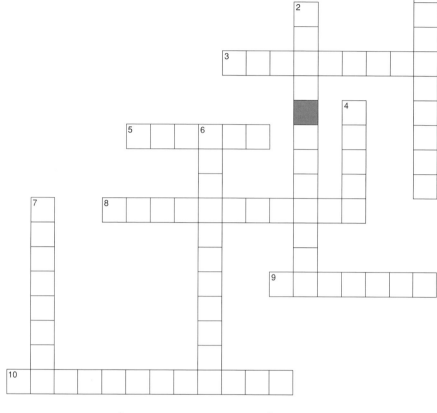

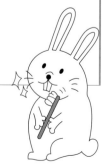

Across

- 3. 治療
- 5. 大臼歯
- 8. 修復
- 9. 詳細
- 10. 歯科矯正学

Down

- 1. 歯痛
- 2. 口腔衛生
- 4. クラウン
- 6. 予約
- 7. 登録する

4 Types of treatment

Listening 1 ⬇14

The clinic will open in 30 minutes. The dentist and the DH are talking about the patients they will see. First, check the words below in the mini dictionary on the next page. Then, listen to 1~7 and number the type of treatment you hear. The first one 1 is done for you.

( ) orthodontic treatment
( ) whitening treatment
( ) partial denture
( ) restoration
(1) cleaning & polishing
( ) permanent filling
( ) extraction

Listening 2 ⬇15

Listen again and write down the sentence you hear.

1. She has an appointment with DH Watanabe for _____ and

   _____.
2. He is going to have some _____ _____.
3. She is having a _____ _____ fitted.
4. He is having some _____ _____.
5. She is having some _____ _____.
6. He is going to have a _____ _____.
7. He is having an _____.

Listening 3 ⬇16

Match the type of treatment 1~5 with the explanations A~E.

1. extraction   ( )
2. orthodontic treatment ( )
3. cleaning & polishing   ( )
4. permanent filling   ( )
5. dentures   ( )

Speaking 1 (D : Dentist)

The dentist is talking to the DH about their schedule.

D : Let's check this morning's schedule.

DH : Okay, we have four patients. First, Ms. Garcia for cleaning and polishing.

D : Okay, and then?

DH : Next is Mr. Diaz. He is going to have some restoration work.

D : Yes, that's right. I remember him.

DH : Then, we have two patients for whitening treatment.

Speaking 2

Target sentences: Talking about patients, types of treatment and appointments

1. She has an appointment with DH Watanabe for cleaning and polishing.
2. He is going to have some restoration work.
3. It will take 20 minutes.
4. Mr. Smith has an appointment at 1 pm.
5. He is having an extraction.

Target vocabulary 17

Match the English words on the left with the Japanese words on the right. Then, listen and check your answers.

1. cleaning a. 充填
2. polishing b. 治療
3. fillings c. 研磨
4. treatment d. 抜歯
5. denture e. 義歯（入れ歯）
6. extraction f. クリーニング

Mini Dictionary

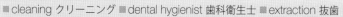
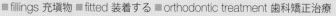
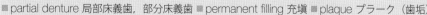

■cleaning クリーニング ■dental hygienist 歯科衛生士 ■extraction 抜歯
■fillings 充填物 ■fitted 装着する ■orthodontic treatment 歯科矯正治療
■partial denture 局部床義歯，部分床義歯 ■permanent filling 充填 ■plaque プラーク（歯垢）
■polishing 研磨 ■remove 取り除く ■replace 取り替える ■restoration 修復
■whitening treatment ホワイトニング治療

5 Questions about medical history

Listening 1 ⬇18

First, check the words below in the mini dictionary on the next page. Then, listen and number the words you hear from 1~10.

( ) illnesses   ( ) hypertension
( ) hospitalized   ( ) dental treatment
( ) suffering from   ( ) sore
( ) medications   ( ) penicillin
( ) painful   ( ) allergic

Listening 2 ⬇19

The DH is helping a patient to fill out a medical history questionnaire. Listen to the patient's answers, circle Yes or No and answer question 10.

Azuma Clinic Medical History Questionnaire

1.	Have you ever had any serious illnesses?	Yes / No
2.	Have you ever been hospitalized?	Yes / No
3.	Are you suffering from hypertension?	Yes / No
4.	Have you seen a doctor recently?	Yes / No
5.	Are you taking any medications?	Yes / No
6.	Are you allergic to any medications?	Yes / No
7.	Have you ever felt bad after dental treatment?	Yes / No
8.	Do your teeth feel sore when you bite on them?	Yes / No
9.	Is it painful when you drink hot, cold or sweet drinks?	Yes / No
10.	When did you last see a dentist?	_____ years ago

Listening 3 ⬇20

Listen to the patient's answers A~E and match them with the questions 1~5.

1. Are you taking any medications?   ( )
2. Are you allergic to any medications?   ( )
3. Have you ever felt bad after dental treatment?   ( )
4. Is it painful when you drink hot, cold or sweet drinks?   ( )
5. When did you last see a dentist?   ( )

Speaking 1

DH : I'd like to ask about your medical history.

PT : Okay. What would you like to know?

DH : Have you ever had any serious illnesses?

PT : No.

DH : Have you ever been hospitalized?

PT : Yes, just once. I broke my leg skiing. I was hospitalized for a week.

DH : Are you suffering from hypertension?

PT : No, my blood pressure is normal.

Speaking 2

Target sentences: Questions about medical history

1. Have you seen a doctor recently?
2. Are you taking any medications?
3. Are you allergic to any medications?
4. Have you ever felt bad after dental treatment?
5. Do your teeth feel sore when you bite on them?
6. Is it painful when you drink hot, cold, or sweet drinks?
7. When did you last see a dentist?

Target vocabulary 21

Listen to someone spelling out these words. Write them down.

1. _____ 7. _____

2. _____ 8. _____

3. _____ 9. _____

4. _____

5. _____

6. _____

Mini Dictionary

■allergic アレルギーの ■anesthetic 麻酔 ■blood pressure 血圧
■cold medicine 風邪薬 ■dizzy めまい ■faint 意識を失う ■healthy 健康的
■hospitalized 入院した ■hypertension 高血圧 ■illness 疾病, 疾患
■medical history 病歴 ■medication 投薬, 服薬 ■painful 痛い, 苦しい
■penicillin ペニシリン ■questionnaire 質問表 ■sore 痛み ■suffering from ～で苦しむ, 悩む

6 Symptoms:
Asking what the problem is
Asking how long the patient has had the problem

Listening 1 ⬇ 22

A patient is telling the DH about a problem. Listen and put the number of the conversation 1~5 in the correct box below.

☐ painful when I chew   ☐ tooth is chipped   ☐ tooth is loose
☐ crown came off   ☐ gums are sensitive   ☐ gums are bleeding
☐ gums are swollen   ☐ have toothache   ☐ filling came out

Listening 2 ⬇ 23

The DH and the dentist are talking about patients and their symptoms. Match the patients with the symptoms.

PATIENTS	SYMPTOMS
1. Mr. Suzuki	a. has toothache
2. Ms. Jones	b. has a loose tooth
3. Joe Sikorski	c. gums are bleeding
4. John Nevara	d. gums are swollen
5. Ms. Tachizawa	e. chipped his front tooth
	f. crown came off

Listening 3 ⬇ 24

How long has the patient had the symptoms? Match each conversation 1~5 with the period of time a~i.

1. (   )
2. (   )
3. (   )
4. (   )
5. (   )

a. since yesterday	g. 24 hours
b. 1 month	h. several hours
c. last week	i. 3 days
d. 2 days	
e. 10 days	
f. 2 or 3 weeks	

Speaking 1

DH : What seems to be the problem?
PT : I have toothache.
DH : I see. When did it start?
PT : Two days ago.
DH : Where does it hurt?
PT : At the back on the lower right.
DH : Okay, let's take a look. Please open wide.

Speaking 2

Target sentences: Asking about symptoms
1. How long have you had this problem?
2. When did the pain start?
3. How long have your gums been swollen?
4. When did your filling come out?
5. How long has this tooth been loose?

Target vocabulary 25

Listen to the Japanese words 1~8 and match them with the English words. Put the number of the word you hear in the brackets.

(　) bleeding
(　) chew
(　) chipped
(　) gums
(　) loose
(　) pain
(　) swollen
(　) symptom

Mini Dictionary

■ bleeding 出血 ■ chew 咀嚼（かむ） ■ crown came off クラウンが取れる
■ denture 義歯 ■ filling came out 充填物が取れる ■ gums 歯肉（歯茎）
■ hard food 硬い食べ物 ■ loose tooth 歯がぐらぐらしている ■ pain 痛み ■ swelling 腫れている
■ symptom 症状 ■ tooth at the back 奥歯 ■ tooth is chipped 歯が欠けた

7 Explaining treatment

 Listening 1 ⬇26

Listen to a DH talking to a patient. The DH is explaining what she is going to do. As you listen, number the steps below from 1~5. Step 1 is done for you.

Examine your teeth and gums	(	)
Note any problems in the chart	(	)
Take some x-rays	(1	)
Check inside your mouth	(	)
Check the x-rays for decay and calculus	(	)

 Listening 2 ⬇27

Now, listen to the rest of the conversation. As you listen, number the steps below from 6~10. Step 6 is done for you.

Remove the hard deposits on your teeth	(	)
Scale your teeth	(6	)
Remove plaque below the gumline	(	)
Polish your teeth	(	)
Floss your teeth	(	)

 Listening 3 ⬇28

Look at the list of verbs in the box. Listen and write down the verb you hear. Some words are used twice.

> remove, scale, examine, note, take, check, polish, floss

1. _____ some x-rays
2. _____ inside your mouth
3. _____ your teeth and gums
4. _____ for decay and calculus
5. _____ your teeth
6. _____ the hard deposits
7. _____ your teeth
8. _____ your teeth
9. _____ any stains

Speaking 1

DH : I'd like to explain about your treatment.
PT : Okay.
DH : First, I'll examine your teeth and gums.
PT : Okay.
DH : Then I'll start to scale your teeth. I'll remove the plaque.
PT : Is that all?
DH : No. I also need to polish your teeth and remove any stains.
PT : How long will it take?
DH : About 40 minutes.

Speaking 2

Target sentences: Explaining treatment

1. I'm going to take some x-rays.
2. I'll check inside your mouth.
3. I'll note any problems in the chart.
4. I'll check the x-rays for decay and calculus.
5. I'll remove the hard deposits from your teeth.
6. I'll remove any stains on your teeth and surface plaque.

Target vocabulary 29

Listen and number the words you hear from 1~9.

( ) gumline   ( ) examine   ( ) calculus
( ) hard deposits ( ) plaque   ( ) polish
( ) chart   ( ) stains   ( ) decay

Mini Dictionary

■calculus 歯石 ■chart 表 ■decay 齲蝕（むし歯）■examine 検査する
■floss デンタルフロスを使う ■gumline（gum line）歯頸線 ■hard deposits 沈着物
■note メモを取る ■plaque プラーク（歯垢）■polish 磨く ■remove 取り除く
■scale スケーリングする ■stain 染み，着色 ■take some x-rays エックス線写真を撮る

Special Listening

Listening to Dental Topics 2

This is a page from a student's notebook. Listen and complete the missing information.

 30

National Smile Week

① (   ) % of people don't know how to brush properly.

② (   ) % of people brush for less than 2 minutes a day.

③ (   ) % of people never floss.

④ (   ) % of people never clean their tongue.

Here are 4 things that people must remember to do.

① (   ) every day.

② (   ) the amount of sugary food and drinks.

③ (   ) the dentist regularly.

④ (   ) healthy snacks like fresh fruit, raw vegetables and cheese.

Crossword Puzzle 2

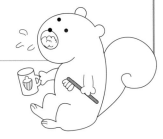

Across
- 3. かむ
- 6. 義歯（入れ歯）
- 7. プラーク（歯垢）
- 8. めまい
- 10. 腫れた
- 11. 歯肉（歯茎）
- 12. 充塡

Down
- 1. 高血圧
- 2. 抜歯
- 4. 出血
- 5. 齲蝕（むし歯）
- 7. 研磨
- 9. 歯石

8 Giving brushing instructions Asking patients questions about brushing

 Listening 1 ⏬31

Look at the pictures below. They are not in the correct order. Listen to the DH telling a patient how to brush. Put the number of the picture 1~5 the DH is talking about in the box on the right of the picture. The first one 1 is done for you.

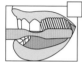   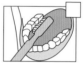 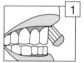

 Listening 2 ⏬32

Listen and complete the sentences by matching 1~6 with a~f.

1. Use a toothbrush with
2. You should replace your toothbrush
3. You should use
4. You should try to
5. After you brush
6. Keep

a. Xylitol in your bag and use it after you snack.
b. soft, nylon, round-ended bristles.
c. use a mouthwash.
d. every 3 or 4 months.
e. floss your teeth every day.
f. toothpaste that contains fluoride.

 Listening 3 ⏬33

The DH is asking patients about brushing. Complete the questions.
1. _____ _____ _____ do you brush your teeth a day?
2. _____ _____ you _____ brush your teeth?
3. How _____ _____ _____ brush your teeth for?
4. _____ _____ _____ brush your teeth?
5. _____ you _____ a _____ or an electric toothbrush?

020 ● 8.GIVING BRUSHING INSTRUCTIONS ASKING PATIENTS QUESTIONS ABOUT BRUSHING   263-00993

Speaking 1

DH : How many times a day do you brush your teeth?
PT : 3 or 4 times a day.
DH : When do you usually brush your teeth?
PT : After meals, and before I go to bed.
DH : How long do you brush your teeth for?
PT : Between 1 and 2 minutes.

Speaking 2

Target sentences: Giving brushing instructions
1. Put the bristles of the brush along the gumline at a 45 degree angle.
2. Brush the outer surface of the teeth.
3. Brush the inner surface of the teeth.
4. Brush behind the front teeth.
5. Brush the biting surface of the teeth.
6. Brush the tongue from back to front.

Target vocabulary ⬇34

Match the English words with the Japanese words. Then, listen and check your answers.

1. bristles	a. 歯頸線
2. gumline	b. 前後
3. outer surface	c. 表層，外面
4. inner surface	d. バクテリア（細菌）
5. biting surface	e. 咬合面
6. bacteria	f. ローリングモーション
7. back and forth	g. 内面
8. rolling motion	h. （ブラシなどの）毛

Mini Dictionary

■ bacteria バクテリア（細菌）■ biting surface 咬合面 ■ bristles （ブラシなどの）毛
■ electric toothbrush 電動歯ブラシ ■ fluoride フッ素 ■ gumline (gum line) 歯頸線
■ inner 内側の ■ manual toothbrush 歯ブラシ（電動でないもの）■ outer 外側の

Giving advice:
Telling patients what they should
or should not do

Listening 1 ⬇ 35

Listen to the DH giving advice. Is it something the patient should or shouldn't do?
Put a check in the correct box and write down the topic.

	Should	Shouldn't	Topic
1.	☐	☐	_____
2.	☐	☐	_____
3.	☐	☐	_____
4.	☐	☐	_____
5.	☐	☐	_____

Listening 2 ⬇ 36

What is the DH talking about?   Select the correct subject (s) a~n.

1. (   )
2. (   )
3. (   )
4. (   )
5. (   )
6. (   )
7. (   )

a. brushing	h. snacking
b. toothpaste	i. plaque
c. toothache	j. whitening
d. fluoride	k. electric toothbrush
e. checkup	l. mouthwash
f. flossing	m. Xylitol
g. smoking	n. toothbrush

Listening 3 ⬇ 37

Listen and complete these sentences.
1. You shouldn't _____.
2. You shouldn't snack or _____ _____ _____.
3. You should brush 3 times a day _____ _____ _____.
4. You should _____ _____ _____ every 6 months.
5. You shouldn't drink too much _____, _____ or _____

_____.

Speaking 1

DH : I'm going to give you some advice.

PT : Okay.

DH : First, smoking. You should give up smoking. It's bad for your teeth and gums.

PT : It's difficult, but I'll try.

DH : Next, snacking. You shouldn't snack too much.

PT : I see.

DH : One more thing. Don't forget to brush after every meal. You should brush for 2 minutes.

Speaking 2

Target sentences: Giving advice

1. You shouldn't smoke.
2. You shouldn't snack.
3. You shouldn't drink sugary drinks.
4. You should brush three times a day.
5. You should floss everyday.
6. You should have a checkup every 6 months.

Target vocabulary 🔽 38

Listen to the sentences A~G. Match them with the English words 1~7.

A. (　　)
B. (　　)
C. (　　)
D. (　　)
E. (　　)
F. (　　)
G. (　　)

1. advice
2. brushing
3. change
4. sugar
5. checkup
6. floss
7. polish

Mini Dictionary

- effective 効果的な - mouthwash マウスウォッシュ - polishing 研磨
- protect 保護する - reduce 減らす - scaling スケーリング
- stained 染みになった，着色した - sugary drinks 糖分を含んだ飲料

Understanding patient questions
How to ask questions

Listening 1 ⬇39

What is the patient asking about? Listen and choose one of the answers from
a ~ l. Before you listen, check the words in the box in the mini dictionary.

1. (   )
2. (   )
3. (   )
4. (   )
5. (   )

a. gums	g. tooth decay
b. gingivitis	h. toothbrush
c. inflammation	i. third molar
d. whiter teeth	j. fluoride
e. Xylitol	k. gum disease
f. plaque	l. sensitive tooth

Listening 2 ⬇40

Listen and complete the questions you hear.
1. Do you _____ _____ _____?
2. _____ _____ _____ you have?
3. Would you like to _____ _____ _____?
4. Is there anything you would _____ _____ _____?
5. _____ _____ _____ any more information?

Listening 3 ⬇41

Match the questions you hear 1~6 with best answers a~f. The first one C is done
for you.

1. (C)
2. (   )
3. (   )
4. (   )
5. (   )
6. (   )

a. Please wait 2 hours before eating or drinking
b. Can you come back next week?
c. Yes, Dr. Suzuki said you need painkillers.
d. No, I need to polish your teeth.
e. At the cashier on the first floor.
f. Your next checkup is in 6 months. We'll send you a recall card.

Speaking 1

DH : Okay, that's the end of today's treatment.
PT : Thank you.
DH : Do you have any questions?
PT : What kind of toothpaste should I use?
DH : You should use toothpaste with fluoride.
PT : Okay, thanks. And, how often should I have a checkup?
DH : Every 6 months. We'll send you a recall card.
PT : Okay, I see.
DH : Is there anything else you'd like to know?
PT : No, I think that's everything.

Speaking 2

Target sentences: Understanding patient questions

1. What causes tooth decay?
2. What causes plaque?
3. What is inflammation?
4. Could you explain about gum disease?
5. How can I get whiter teeth?

Target vocabulary 42

Listen to the English words and match them with the Japanese words a~g.

1. (　　)
2. (　　)
3. (　　)
4. (　　)
5. (　　)
6. (　　)
7. (　　)

| a. プラーク（歯垢） |
| b. 炎症 |
| c. 染み，着色 |
| d. 歯周病 |
| e. フッ素 |
| f. 齲蝕（むし歯） |
| g. より白い歯 |

Mini Dictionary

■fluoride フッ素 ■gum disease 歯周病 ■gums 歯肉（歯茎）■inflammation 炎症 ■look dark 汚くみえる ■medicine 薬 ■plaque プラーク（歯垢）■sensitive tooth 知覚過敏 ■stains 染み，着色 ■third molar 第三大臼歯（親知らず）■tooth decay 齲蝕（むし歯）

Giving advice to a patient who is going to have a tooth extracted

Listening 1 📥43

Match the sentences on the left 1~5 with those on the right a~g.

1. You should avoid (　　　).
2. If your gum starts to bleed, (　　　).
3. If the bleeding doesn't stop, (　　　).
4. On the day after the extraction, (　　　).
5. Don't forget to (　　　).

a. brush your teeth
b. hot or spicy food and drinks
c. please contact us
d. come back a week later
e. rinse your mouth with hot, salt water
f. take some aspirin
g. bite firmly on a sterile gauze pad

Listening 2 📥44

Listen to the sentences and circle the correct information.

1. Dr. Watanabe will need to extract (a tooth / 2 teeth / 3 teeth).
2. You will probably experience some (discomfort / pain / bleeding).
3. I'd like to give you some general (information / advice / suggestions).
4. Also, avoid smoking and (chewing gum / alcohol / hot drinks).
5. You should change the pad every (20 / 25 / 35) minutes.

Listening 3 📥45

Listen to these words. Are they singular or plural ? Circle the word you hear.

1. tooth ／ teeth
2. drink ／ drinks
3. pad ／ pads
4. appointment ／ appointments
5. extraction ／ extractions

Speaking 1

DH : Dr. Watanabe will need to extract a tooth. He asked me to give you some advice.
PT : Okay. Thank you.
DH : You should avoid hot or spicy food and drinks. Also, avoid smoking and alcohol.
PT : Okay, I've got that.
DH : If your gum starts to bleed, bite firmly on a sterile gauze pad. Change the pad every 20 minutes.
PT : Okay, I understand.

 Speaking 2

Target sentences: Talking to a patient who is going to have a tooth extracted
1. After the extraction, you will probably experience some pain and discomfort.
2. If the bleeding doesn't stop, please contact us.
3. Rinse your mouth with hot salt water or use an antiseptic mouthwash.
4. Don't forget you need to come back a week later.
5. Don't worry. It'll be okay.

Target vocabulary ⬇️46

Listen to the sentences A~G and match them with the English words 1~7.

A. (   )
B. (   )
C. (   )
D. (   )
E. (   )
F. (   )
G. (   )

1. orthodontic treatment
2. extract
3. pain
4. discomfort
5. avoid
6. sterile gauze pad
7. rinse

Mini Dictionary

■bite かむ ■discomfort 不快 ■extract a tooth 抜歯をする ■extraction 抜歯
■gauze ガーゼ ■rinse 洗浄する ■sterile 滅菌した，滅菌された

Telling a patient about medicine
Giving directions to a pharmacy

Listening 1 📥47

Listen and circle the correct information.
1. Mr. Smith will have to take (2 / 3 / 4) kinds of medicine.
2. Antibiotics will prevent (pain / infection / tooth decay).
3. He should take (1 / 2 / 3) tablet(s) (1 / 2 / 3) time(s) a day for
   (1 / 2 / 3) day(s).
4. He should take the painkillers (before / after) the anesthetic wears off.
5. With painkillers, he must not take more than (1 / 2 / 3 / 4) tablet(s) a day.

Listening 2 📥48

Listen and complete the grid.

	How many tablets?	How many times a day?	For how many days?	When?
1				
2				
3				
4				

Listening 3 📥49

The patient is asking for directions to a pharmacy. Listen and circle the correct location.

1.

reception | cashier
main entrance
o o o o o o
o o o o o o

2.

reception | office
elevator

3.

hospital | post office | gas st.
dental clinic | hamburger shop

Speaking 1

DH : Here is your medicine. You have 2 kinds of medicine.
PT : Two kinds?
DH : Yes, antibiotics and painkillers.
PT : Okay.
DH : I'll explain how to take them. First, antibiotics. Take 1 tablet 3 times a day after meals.
PT : Okay, I've got that.
DH : Take the painkillers before the anesthetic wears off.

Speaking 2

Target sentences: Telling a patient about medicine   Giving directions to a pharmacy

1. I need to tell you about your medicine.
2. Antibiotics prevent infection.
3. It is very important to finish all the tablets.
4. Take 2 tablets 3 times a day after meals.
5. The pharmacy is on the right next to the cashier.
6. There is a pharmacy 2 or 3 minutes from here.

Target vocabulary 50

Listen to the Japanese words A~H and match them with English words 1~8. Then, write down the Japanese words.

A. (   ) _____
B. (   ) _____
C. (   ) _____
D. (   ) _____
E. (   ) _____
F. (   ) _____
G. (   ) _____
H. (   ) _____

1.	antibiotics
2.	painkillers
3.	infection
4.	anesthetic
5.	wear off
6.	twice a day
7.	three times a day
8.	medicine

Mini Dictionary

■antibiotics 抗生物質 ■anesthetic 麻酔 ■cashier 会計
■pain killers 痛み止め，鎮痛剤 ■pharmacy 薬局 ■wear off （薬が）きれる

Explaining where to pay, the cost of treatment and the price of dental products

Listening 1 🔽 51

Listen to the DH explaining where to pay. Choose the correct expression a~g from the box on the right.

1. (   )
2. (   )
3. (   )
4. (   )
5. (   )

a. at the reception
b. on the first floor
c. on the third floor
d. in the waiting area
e. at the window on the left
f. next to the reception
g. the window in the middle

Listening 2 🔽 52

How much does the patient need to pay? Listen and select the correct amount a~j from the box on the right.

1. (   )
2. (   )
3. (   )
4. (   )
5. (   )

a. ¥5,950	f. ¥678
b. ¥11,150	g. ¥687
c. ¥15,500	h. ¥1,150
d. ¥150,000	i. ¥5,850
e. ¥13,975	j. ¥31,975

Listening 3 🔽 53

Listen to the DH giving advice. Circle the 5 things the DH recommended the patient to buy. How much do they cost? Draw a line.

PRODUCTS
1. gauze pads
2. toothbrush
3. painkillers
4. fluoride toothpaste
5. cotton pads
6. interdental brushes
7. Xylitol gum
8. dental floss
9. mouthwash
10. dental mirror

PRICE
a. ¥1,344
b. ¥9,931
c. ¥733
d. ¥295
e. ¥5,500
f. ¥378
g. ¥418
h. ¥523
i. ¥155
j. ¥313

Speaking 1

PT : Excuse me, where do I pay?
DH : You can pay on the first floor.
PT : How do I get there?
DH : Take the elevator. You can pay next to the reception.
PT : Thank you very much.
DH : Take a seat in the waiting room. The receptionist will call your name.
PT : Okay, I've got that.

Speaking 2

Target sentences: Explaining where to pay, how much to pay, and recommending dental products
1. You can pay at reception.
2. The receptionist will call your name.
3. Go down to the first floor. You can pay there.
4. The cost of today's treatment is ¥5,850.
5. That's ¥1,150, please.
6. You need to have some dental floss.
7. Why don't you buy some mouthwash?

Target vocabulary 54

Listen and number the words you hear.
(　) reception
(　) receptionist
(　) pay
(　) treatment
(　) dental hygiene products

Mini Dictionary

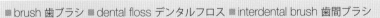

■ brush 歯ブラシ ■ dental floss デンタルフロス ■ interdental brush 歯間ブラシ
■ mouthwash マウスウォッシュ ■ products 製品 ■ reception 受付
■ receptionist 受付係 ■ window 窓口

14 What do dental hygienists need for the job?
What's a typical day for a DH?

Listening 1 55

Listen to this interview with Carol, a DH from California. Circle the correct information and complete sentence 2.

1. Carol has been a dental hygienist for (2 / 12 / 20) years.
2. She said the most important part of her job is to teach people how to
_____ and _____.

Listening 2 56

What do dental hygienists need for the job? Listen and choose 4 things from a~f.

1. You need to be (   )
2. You need to be (   )
3. You need to be (   )
4. You need to be (   )

a. kind to patients.
b. interested in science.
c. polite and cheerful.
d. able to communicate well with patients.
e. good with your hands.
f . patient.

Listening 3 57

Carol is talking about a typical day for a DH. Listen and complete these sentences by choosing words from the box below.

1. I examine the patient's _____ and _____.
2. I write this information _____ for the dentist to see later.
3. I _____ and check for tooth decay and calculus.
4. I _____ the patient's teeth.
5. I remove any _____ on the teeth.
6. I also remove any _____ below the _____.
7. Then, I _____ the teeth to remove _____ and _____.

surface plaque	polish	calculus
teeth	on the chart	scale
stains	gumline	take x-rays
gums	plaque	

Speaking 1

(Int : Interviewer)

Int : How long have you been a DH?

DH : For more than 20 years.

Int : What do dental hygienists need for the job?

DH : Well, 4 things. You need to be interested in science. You need to be able to communicate well. You need to be patient. You need to be good with your hands.

Int : Could you tell me about a typical day for a DH?

DH : Sure. I arrive at the clinic at 8:30. I check …

Speaking 2

Target sentences: Talking about a typical day

1. I start with an intra-oral and extra-oral examination.
2. I examine the patient's teeth and gums.
3. I write this information on the chart.
4. I take x-rays and check for tooth decay and calculus.
5. I scale the teeth to remove any hard deposits.
6. I remove plaque that is below the gumline.
7. Then, I polish the teeth to remove stains and surface plaque.

Target vocabulary 58

Listen to the Japanese words and match them with the English words 1~10.
Then, write down the Japanese words.

A. (　)　_____
B. (　)　_____
C. (　)　_____
D. (　)　_____
E. (　)　_____
F. (　)　_____
G. (　)　_____
H. (　)　_____
I. (　)　_____
J. (　)　_____

1. good with your hands
2. intra-oral
3. extra-oral
4. calculus
5. decay
6. setting up the room
7. polish
8. remove surface plaque
9. chart
10. scale

Mini Dictionary

■ brush 歯ブラシ ■ calculus 歯石 ■ communicate with 〜 意思の疎通をはかる
■ dental hygienist 歯科衛生士 ■ good with your hands 手が器用である
■ science 科学 ■ typical day 典型的な一日

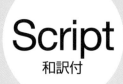

1. Have you visited us before?

 Listening 1 📥 01

❶

DH: Good morning. Azuma Dental Clinic. DH Suzuki speaking.

PT: Good morning. I'd like to make an appointment.

DH: Have you visited us before?

PT: No, this is my first time.

DH: So, you need to register. First, let me take some details. Could I have your name, please?

PT: Sure. It's Bill Smith.

DH: Do you have Japanese health insurance?

PT: Yes, I do.

- -

DH: おはようございます．アズマデンタルクリニックです．歯科衛生士の鈴木がお受けいたします．

PT: おはようございます．予約をしたいのですが.

DH: 以前にこちらに通院されたことはございますか？

PT: いいえ，今回がはじめてです．

DH: では登録をしたいと思います．いくつかおうかがいしたいのですが，まずお名前をおっしゃっていただけますか？

PT: はい．ビル・スミスと申します．

DH: 日本の健康保険証をお持ちですか？

PT: はい，持っています．

- -

❷

DH: Nishi Dental Clinic. How may I help you?

PT: I just moved to this area and I'd like to register with a dentist.

DH: So, you are a new patient.

PT: That's right.

DH: First, let me take some details. Could I have your name, please? And, could I also have your address, and telephone number?

- -

DH: はい，ニシデンタルクリニックです．ご用件はなんでしょうか？

PT: この地域に引っ越して来たばかりなのですが，歯科医院にかかりたいのです．

DH: では，初診の方ですね？

PT: その通りです．

DH: では，いくつかおうかがいしたいのですが，まずお名前をおっしゃっていただけますか？ご住所とお電話番号もお願いします．

- -

❸

DH: Higashi Dental Clinic. DH Watanabe speaking.

PT: Hi. I got a recall card yesterday. Do I need to make an appointment?

DH: Yes, registered patients with recall cards need an appointment. When can you come in?

PT: Well, I'm busy this week, but next week is okay.

DH: Just a moment. I'll check the schedule.

- -

DH: ヒガシデンタルクリニックです．歯科衛生士の渡辺がお受けいたします．

PT: こんにちは．昨日，定期検診のハガキが届いたのですが，予約をする必要はありますか？

DH: はい，定期検診の患者さんも予約が必要です．いつがよろしいですか？

PT: えー，今週は忙しいのですが，来週なら大丈夫です．

DH: 少々お待ちください．予定を確認してみます．

- -

❹

DH: Good morning. Sakura dental clinic. How can I help you?

PT: My name's John Smith. I'd like to make an appointment to have my teeth cleaned.

DH: Mr. Smith, are you registered with us?

PT: Yes, I am.

DH: Do you have Japanese health insurance?

263-00993

PT: Yes, I do.

- -

DH: おはようございます. サクラデンタルクリニックです. いかがいたしましたか?

PT: ジョン・スミスと申します. 歯のクリーニングのために予約を入れたいのですが.

DH: スミス様ですね. こちらにいらしたことはございますか?

PT: はい.

DH: 日本の健康保険証をお持ちですか?

PT: はい, 持っています.

❺

DH: Good afternoon. Azuma Dental Clinic, DH Suzuki speaking.

PT: Hi. My name is Steve Jenkins. I have an appointment sometime this week to have my teeth cleaned. I'm sorry, I forgot the day and the time. Could you check it for me, please?

DH: Yes, of course. Could I have your name again, please?

PT: Yes, it's Jenkins. That's J-E-N-K-I-N-S.

DH: Mr. Jenkins, I'm just checking our computer records. Yes, your appointment is for Thursday this week with DH Watanabe at 10:30am. Please bring your health insurance card.

PT: Yes, of course. Now I remember. Thursday 10:30. Sorry to have troubled you. See you on Thursday.

- -

DH: こんにちは, アズマデンタルクリニックです. 歯科衛生士の鈴木がお受けいたします.

PT: もしもし, スティーブ・ジェンキンスと申します. 歯のクリーニングのために今週予約を入れていたはずなのですが, 日時を忘れてしまいました. 確認していただけませんか?

DH: はい, もう一度お名前をおっしゃってください.

PT: はい, ジェンキンスと申します. J-E-N-K-I-N-S です.

DH: ジェンキンスさんですね. いま, コンピュータで記録を調べています. はい, 今週木曜日の午前10:30 に歯科衛生士の渡辺担当で予約が入っています. 保険証をお持ちのうえお越しください.

PT: わかりました. あ, いま思い出しました. 木曜日の午前10:30 ですね. ご迷惑をおかけしてすみません. では木曜日にうかがいます.

 Listening 2 02

1. Have you visited us before?
2. Could I have your name, please?
3. Could you spell that, please?
4. When can you come in?
5. How about Tuesday or Wednesday next week at about 5:30?
6. Do you have Japanese health insurance?

A. Sure, it's S-M-I-T-H.
B. Sure, it's Bill Smith.
C. No, this is my first time.
D. Tuesday at 5:30 would be fine.
E. I'm busy this week, but I could make it next week.
F. Japanese health insurance. Yes, I do.

- -

1. 以前こちらにいらっしゃったことはございますか?
2. お名前をお教えください.
3. 綴りをお教えください.
4. いつこちらにいらっしゃることができますか?
5. 来週火曜日か水曜日の5：30 はいかがでしょうか?
6. 日本の健康保険証をお持ちですか?

A. はい. S-M-I-T-H です.
B. はい. ビル・スミスと申します.
C. いいえ, 今回がはじめてです.
D. 火曜日の5：30 なら大丈夫です.
E. 今週は忙しいですが, 来週なら都合がつけられます.
F. 日本の健康保険証ですね. はい, 持ってます.

 Listening 3 03

1. recall card
2. clinic
3. details
4. dentist
5. appointment
6. teeth

- -

1. 定期検診のハガキ

2. 診療所
3. 詳細
4. 歯科医師
5. 予約
6. 歯

2. Taking a patient's name, address, telephone number Filling out a registration card

Listening 1 05

1

DH: Could I have your name, please?
PT: It's Hughes. Bill Hughes.
DH: Could you spell that, please?
PT: Sure. It's H-U-G-H-E-S. That's my family name.
DH: Just a moment. H-U-G-H-E-S. And your first name is Bill, right?
PT: That's right.
DH: Okay, Mr. Hughes. I've got that. Thank you.

DH: お名前をおっしゃっていただけますか？
PT: ヒューズと申します．ビル・ヒューズです．
DH: 綴りをお願いします．
PT: はい，H-U-G-H-E-S です．それが，私の苗字です．
DH: 少々お待ちください．H-U-G-H-E-S さんですね．下のお名前はビルさんでよろしいですね？
PT: その通りです．
DH: はい，ヒューズ様 かしこまりました．ありがとうございます．

2

DH: I need to take your details. What is your name?
PT: Peter Cowley.
DH: Would you mind spelling that?
PT: No, not at all. It's C-O-W-L-E-Y. And my first name is Peter.
DH: Okay, Mr. Cowley. I've got that. Thanks.

DH: いくつかおうかがいしたいのですが，お名前は何ですか？
PT: ピーター・カウリーです．
DH: 綴りをおっしゃっていただけませんか？
PT: はい，C-O-W-L-E-Y です．下の名前はピーターです．
DH: はい，カウリー様 かしこまりました．ありがとうございます．

3

DH: Could you fill out this registration card, please?
PT: Yes, of course. Oh, it's in Japanese. I'm afraid I can't read Japanese.
DH: Okay. I'll help you. Could I have your family name?
PT: It's Davies.
DH: Is that D-A-V-I-E-S?
PT: Yes, that's right.
DH: And, what's your first name?
PT: James.
DH: Okay, Mr. Davies. And how old are you?
PT: 38.
DH: Could I have your address, please?
PT: Sure, it's・・・

DH: この診療申込書に記入してください.
PT: はい, わかりました. あっ, これは日本語ですね. すみませんが, 私は日本語が読めません.
DH: かしこまりました. お手伝いしましょう. 苗字を教えてください.
PT: デービスです.
DH: D-A-V-I-E-S ですか?
PT: はい, その通りです.
DH: では, 下のお名前は何ですか?
PT: ジェイムズです.
DH: かしこまりました, デービス様. おいくつですか?
PT: 38 歳です.
DH: ご住所を教えてください.
PT: はい. 住所は・・・

DH: Could I have your family name, please?
PT: Yes, it's Boyd.
DH: Could you spell that, please?
PT: Yes. It's B-O-Y-D.
DH: What's your first name?
PT: Dave.

DH: 苗字を教えてください.
PT: はい, ボイドです.
DH: 綴りを教えてください.
PT: はい, B-O-Y-D です.
DH: 下のお名前は何ですか?
PT: デイブです.

DH: Could I have your name, please?
PT: It's Jones. Sarah Jones.
DH: Could you spell that?
PT: Sure. It's J-O-N-E-S. That's my family name.
DH: J-O-N-E-S. And your first name is Sarah, right?
PT: That's right.
DH: Thank you. Could you fill out this registration card, please?

DH: お名前を教えてください.
PT: ジョーンズです. セーラ・ジョーンズです.

DH: 綴りを教えてください.
PT: はい, J-O-N-E-S です. それが, 苗字です.
DH: J-O-N-E-S さんですね. 下のお名前はセーラさんでよろしいですね?
PT: その通りです.
DH: ありがとうございます. この診療申込書に記入してください.

Listening 2　06

DH: Could I have your name, please?
PT: Yes, of course. It's Nevara. That's N-E-V-A-R-A. My first name is John.

DH: お名前をお願いします.
PT: はい, ネバラです. N-E-V-A-R-A です. 下の名前はジョンです.

DH: Could you spell your name, please?
PT: Sure. It's Williams. That's W-I-L-L-I-A-M-S. My first name is Paul.

DH: お名前の綴りをお教えください.
PT: はい, ウイリアムズです. W-I-L-L-I-A-M-S です. 下の名前はポールです.

DH: And, what's your family name?
PT: Sikorski. That's S-I-K-O-R-S-K-I. My first name is Jim.

DH: では苗字をお願いします.
PT: シコルスキーです. S-I-K-O-R-S-K-I です. 下の名前はジムです.

PT: My first name is Dan, and my family name is Waldhoff. I'll spell that for you. It's W-A-L-D-H-O-F-F.
DH: Okay, I've got that. Thank you.

DH: 下の名前はダンです．苗字はワルドホフです．綴り
　　を言います．W-A-L-D-H-O-F-F です．
PT: かしこまりました．ありがとうございます．

PT: My family name is Wright. That's W-R-I-G-
　　H-T.
DH: And your first name?
PT: Cameron.
DH: Okay. I've got that. Thank you.

- -

PT: 苗字はライトです．W-R-I-G-H-T です．
DH: 下のお名前は？
DH: キャメロンです．
PT: かしこまりました．ありがとうございます．

Listening 3 07

DH: Let me help you fill out this registration
　　card.
PT: Thank you.
DH: So, your first name is John.
PT: That's right.
DH: What's your family name?
PT: Richards
DH: Could you spell that please?
PT: Yes, it's R-I-C-H-A-R-D-S.
DH: Thank you, Mr. Richards. And how old are
　　you?
PT: I'm 38.
DH: 38. What is your address?
PT: It's Minato City, Higashi 3-5-207.
DH: Higashi 3-5-207. Thanks. And, could
　　I have your telephone number?
PT: Sure. It's 08034018783.
DH: Thanks. I've got that. Could you wait here,
　　please? Dr. Suzuki will be with you soon.

- -

DH: この診療申込書に記入するのをお手伝いしましょ
　　う．
PT: ありがとうございます．
DH: 下のお名前はジョンさんですね．
PT: その通りです．
DH: 苗字は何ですか？
PT: リチャーズです．

DH: 綴りを教えてください．
PT: はい，R-I-C-H-A-R-D-S です．
DH: ありがとうございます，リチャーズ様　おいくつで
　　しょうか？
PT: 38 歳です．
DH: 38 歳ですね．では，ご住所を教えてください．
PT: 港市東 3-5-207 です．
DH: 東 3-5-207 ですね．ありがとうございます．お電
　　話番号をお願いします．
PT: はい．080-3401-8783 です．
DH: はい，ありがとうございます．かしこまりました．
　　ここで少々お待ちください．鈴木先生がすぐに参り
　　ます．

- -

Target vocabulary 08

1. 記入する
2. 診療申込書
3. 苗字
4. 名前
5. 電話番号
6. 住所

3 Making appointments:
Days, dates, times

Listening 1 📥 09

❶

DH: Dr. Suzuki wants to check your new
　　crown. So, we need to make another
　　appointment. When would be convenient,
　　Mr. Williams?
PT: I'm free on Tuesdays. So, could I come in
　　next Tuesday?
DH: Let me check. That would be Tuesday,
　　March the 20th. What time would suit you?
PT: The earlier, the better.
DH: Okay. How about 9am?
PT: That's fine.
DH: Okay. So, that's Tuesday, March the 20th
　　at 9am.

- -

DH: 鈴木先生があなたの新しいクラウンを検査したいそ
　　うです．次の予約をしていただきたいのですが，ウ

イリアムズ様はいつご都合がよろしいですか？

PT: 火曜日が都合がよいです．来週の火曜日に来てもよいですか？

DH: 確認します．3月20日の火曜日ですね．何時がよいでしょうか？

PT: 早い時間がよいです．

DH: かしこまりました．では午前9時はどうでしょうか？

PT: 大丈夫です．

DH: かしこまりました．では3月20日火曜日の午前9時にお願いします．

- -

DH: We need to arrange another appointment. Dr. Suzuki said you need some restoration on one of your molars. He said you have some decay. When can you come in, Mr. Jones?

PT: I'm away for the rest of this week on business. And next Monday is a national holiday. How about next Wednesday? It's April the 10th.

DH: Wednesday is fine, but Dr. Suzuki is busy in the morning. How about the afternoon?

PT: That's no problem. I'm free all afternoon.

DH: Okay. So, let's make it 3pm next Wednesday, which is April the 10th.

- -

DH: 次の予約をお願いしたいと思います．奥歯の修復治療をしなければいけないと鈴木先生がおっしゃっています．先生によると，むし歯があるようです．ジョーンズさんはいつご都合がよろしいでしょうか？

PT: 今週は出張で出かけてしまいます．来週の月曜日は祝日ですもんね．来週の水曜日はどうでしょうか？4月10日です．

DH: 水曜日は大丈夫ですが，鈴木先生は午前中は予約でいっぱいです．午後はいかがでしょうか？

PT: 大丈夫です．午後はずっと時間があります．

DH: かしこまりました．では，4月10日水曜日の午後3時にしましょう．

- -

3

DH: For this treatment, Ms. Chang, you will need to come in once a week for three

or four weeks. Can we make the first appointment sometime early next week?

PT: You mean Monday or Tuesday?

DH: That's right.

PT: Well, I'm out of town on Monday, so it will have to be Tuesday. Is that the 17th?

DH: Just a moment. I'll check. No, it's the 18th. December the 18th. What time is convenient for you?

PT: How about 3:30?

DH: I'm sorry, but the dentist has a patient then. Could you make it a bit later?

PT: 4:30 would be okay for me.

DH: Okay. So that is Tuesday, December the 18th at 4:30.

- -

DH: チャンさん，この治療では3〜4週間は週に一度通院していただく必要があります．最初の予約を来週のはじめに入れたいのですが，いかがでしょうか？

PT: それは月曜日か火曜日ということですね？

DH: そうです．

PT: えーと，私は月曜日は出かけますので，火曜日がよいです．17日でしたっけ？

DH: 少々お待ちください．確認します．いいえ，18日ですね．12月18日です．何時がご都合よろしいですか？

PT: 3：30でどうでしょうか？

DH: 申し訳ございませんが，その時間はほかの患者さんがいらっしゃいます．もう少し遅い時間でどうでしょうか？

PT: 4：30なら大丈夫です．

DH: かしこまりました．では，12月18日火曜日の4：30にお願いします．

- -

4

DH: Okay, Ms.Clinton. Dr. Suzuki said your orthodontic treatment is going well. But he is worried about your oral hygiene. When you are wearing braces, sometimes it is difficult to brush properly and plaque builds up in some places. He said you should make an appointment to see a dental hygienist. When can you come in?

PT: How about Friday next week?

DH: Okay, so that is June the 17th. Would 7:30

pm be okay?

PT: Yes, that's fine.

DH: ではクリントンさん、鈴木先生がおっしゃるには、歯科矯正治療はうまくいっているようです。しかし、先生はあなたの口腔衛生を心配しています。歯列矯正装置を着けていると、しっかりと歯磨きをすることが難しくなり、場所によっては歯垢がついてしまうからです。そこで歯科衛生士の予約を入れられることをおすすめしていますが、いつなら来院できますか？

PT: 来週の金曜日はどうでしょうか？

DH: かしこまりました。6月17日ですね。午後7：30でよいでしょうか？

PT: はい、かまいません。

DH: We need to arrange another appointment.

PT: Okay.

DH: How about April the 10th?

PT: Is that Thursday or Friday?

DH: It's Friday.

PT: That's fine.

DH: Is 2pm good for you?

PT: Yes, that's great.

DH: 次の予約を入れていただきたいのですが。

PT: わかりました。

DH: 4月10日はどうでしょうか？

PT: それは木曜日ですか、それとも金曜日ですか？

DH: 金曜日です。

PT: 大丈夫です。

DH: 午後2：00でご都合よろしいですか？

PT: はい、大丈夫です。

---

1. So your next appointment, Mr. Smith, is on May the 30th at 10:30.
2. Would June the 15th be okay for you?
3. Dr. Suzuki is free on May the 6th.
4. How about October the 19th?
5. Your next appointment is in 2 weeks. It's December the 14th.

---

1. では、今度の予約はですね、スミスさん、5月30日の10：30です。
2. 6月15日でよろしいですか？
3. 鈴木先生は5月6日があいています。
4. 10月19日はどうでしょうか？
5. 今度の予約は2週間後です。12月14日です。

---

1. Okay. Your next appointment is at 3:15.
2. Okay. See you tomorrow at 8pm.
3. I'm free on Monday at 9:15.
4. The clinic opens at 8:45.
5. So, that's 3:20. No, sorry, I meant 2:20.

---

1. かしこまりました。あなたの次の予約は3：15です。
2. かしこまりました。では午後8：00にお会いしましょう。
3. 月曜日の9：15なら時間があります。
4. 診療時間は8：45からです。
5. では、3：20でお願いします。いや、すみません、2：20です。

---

1. クラウン
2. 修復
3. 臼歯
4. 歯科矯正治療
5. 口腔衛生
6. 歯列矯正装置
7. 正しく磨く
8. 歯科衛生

Special Listening— 13
Listening to dental topics 1

Here is some dental data from the UK. First, oral health problems. Do you know how many people visit their dentist with toothache every year? The answer is about 5 million. That's a lot of people.

What about fillings? How many fillings do adults have? Well, about 30 per cent of adults have

12 or more fillings. 12 fillings. That's a lot.
Okay the next topic is oral health routine. How often do people brush their teeth? We all know that you should brush 3 times daily. But, the survey showed 1 in 5 people brush their teeth less than twice a day. Less than twice a day is not enough.

Here's another question. How often do people change their toothbrush? Most adults in the UK only change their toothbrush once a year. Again this is not enough.

And here is the last point. In the UK, 39 per cent of people use an electric toothbrush.

これは英国の歯科についてのデータです．まず，はじめに，口腔保健に関してです．毎年，歯痛で歯科医院を訪れる人が何人くらいいるか知っていますか？ 答えはおよそ500万人です．たくさんいますね．

では，充填物についてはどうでしょうか．成人ではどれくらい充填物を入れていると思いますか？ およそ成人の30%が12カ所以上の充填物を入れています．12ですよ．これも多いですね．

次のトピックは，口腔保健の習慣についてです．英国人はどのくらいの頻度で歯を磨いているのでしょうか？ 私たちは，1日に3回は磨くべきだということをみんなが知っていますよね．しかし，調査によると，5人に1人は1日に2回以下しか磨いていません．1日に2回以下では十分とはいえませんね．

もう1つ問題です．英国人はどのくらいの頻度で歯ブラシを替えているでしょうか？ 英国の成人の多くは，1年に1回しか歯ブラシを替えていません．これもまた十分とはいえませんね．

最後にもう1つお知らせします．英国では39%の人が電動歯ブラシを使っています．

4　Types of treatment

Listening 1 14

1. Okay, let's just check through the patients we have this morning. At 9 am, we have Ms. Sukarno. She has an appointment with DH Watanabe for cleaning and polishing. If you have any problems, let me know.
2. After that is Mr. Morton. He is going to

have some restoration work. Dr. Suzuki will replace some old fillings with new ones.
3. At 10:00, we have Joe Sikorski and his mother. Joe is 12 years old. He is having some orthodontic treatment. It should only take about half an hour. I'm worried about his oral hygiene. I want him to make an appointment with the dental hygienist. Can you talk to his mother about that?
4. Then, we have Ms. Williams. She is having a partial denture fitted. It will take 20 minutes.
5. Ms. Suzuki is coming in at 11:00. She is having some whitening treatment.
6. Mr. Smith has an appointment at 11:30. He is having a permanent filling.
7. The last patient before lunch is Mr. Salisbury. He is having an extraction. I'd like you to give him some advice on what to do after the extraction.

1. それでは，今日の午前中に予約が入っている患者さんを確認しましょう．9：00はスカルノ様です．歯科衛生士の渡辺さんが担当で，歯のクリーニングと研磨の予約が入っています．何か問題がありましたら教えてください．
2. その後はモートンさんです．修復治療を行う予定です．鈴木先生が古くなった充填物を新しいものと取り替えます．
3. 10：00には，ジョー・シコルスキー君とお母さんがいらっしゃいます．ジョー君は12歳で，歯科矯正治療のために来ます．30分くらいで済むでしょう．彼の口腔衛生が心配です．歯科衛生士の予約を取るべきだと思います．そのことをお母さんに話してくれませんか．
4. それから，ウイリアムズさんです．部分床義歯を装着します．20分くらいでしょう．
5. 11：00には鈴木さんが来院されます．彼女はホワイトニング治療を行います．
6. 11：30にはスミスさんの予約が入っています．充填の予定です．
7. 午前中の最後の患者さんはソールズベリーさんです．彼は抜歯をします．抜歯後のアドバイスをしてあげてください．

Listening 2 15

1. She has an appointment with DH Watanabe

for cleaning and polishing.
2. He is going to have some restoration work.
3. She is having a partial denture fitted.
4. He is having some orthodontic treatment.
5. She is having some whitening treatment.
6. He is going to have a permanent filling.
7. He is having an extraction.

---

1. 彼女は歯のクリーニングと研磨の予定で，歯科衛生士の渡辺さん担当で予約が入っています．
2. 彼は修復治療を行う予定です．
3. 彼女は部分床義歯を装着します．
4. 彼は歯科矯正治療を行います．
5. 彼女はホワイトニング治療を行います．
6. 彼は充填を行う予定です．
7. 彼は抜歯をします．

Listening 3 16

A. In this treatment, you make a patient's teeth straight. You use wires called a brace. Some children have this treatment.
B. This treatment is done by a dental hygienist. The DH removes the plaque.
C. People with no natural teeth need false teeth.
D. If a tooth has too much decay, it must be taken out.
E. The dentist drills a tooth to remove decay then puts in a filling.

A. この治療では，患者さんの歯をまっすぐにします．歯列矯正装置としてワイヤーを使います．児童たちはこの治療を行うことがあります．
B. この治療は歯科衛生士が担当します．歯科衛生士は歯垢を取り除いてくれます．
C. 天然歯がない人には義歯が必要です．
D. むし歯がたくさんあったら，抜くこともあります．
E. 歯科医師はむし歯を取り除くために歯を削り，充填物を入れます．

Target vocabulary 17

1. cleaning クリーニング
2. polishing 研磨
3. fillings 充填
4. treatment 治療

---

5. denture 義歯（入れ歯）
6. extraction 抜歯

5 Questions about medical history

Listening 1 18

1. hypertension
2. illnesses
3. sore
4. medications
5. painful
6. hospitalized
7. dental treatment
8. suffering from
9. penicillin
10. allergic

---

1. 高血圧
2. 疾病，疾患
3. 痛み
4. 投薬，服薬
5. 痛い，苦しい
6. 入院した
7. 歯科治療
8. ～で苦しむ，悩む
9. ペニシリン
10. アレルギーの

Listening 2 19

DH: I'd like to ask you about your medical history.
PT: My medical history. Okay. What would you like to know?
DH: I have a short questionnaire here. It has ten questions. I'll just read through the questions with you. Could you circle 'Yes' or 'No' on the questionnaire?
PT: Sure.
DH: Question one. Have you ever had any serious illnesses?
PT: Serious illnesses. No. I've always been very healthy.

DH: Have you ever been hospitalized?

PT: Yes, just once. I broke my leg skiing. I was hospitalized for a week.

DH: I see. Are you suffering from hypertension?

PT: Hypertension? Sorry, what's that?

DH: It means high blood pressure. Are you suffering from high blood pressure?

PT: No, my blood pressure is normal.

DH: Have you seen a doctor recently?

PT: No, I'm in good health. I haven't seen a doctor for several years.

DH: Well, that's great. Are you taking any medications?

PT: No.

DH: Are you allergic to any medications?

PT: No, I'm not.

DH: Have you ever felt bad after dental treatment?

PT: Felt bad. Sorry? What do you mean?

DH: Well, after treatment, have you ever felt faint or dizzy?

PT: Faint or dizzy. No, I've never had any problems like that.

DH: Do your teeth feel sore when you bite on them?

PT: Yes, they do. Particularly, the one at the back, on the lower right.

DH: I'll make a note of that in the chart. The dentist will check it. Is it painful when you drink hot, cold or sweet drinks?

PT: Yes, sometimes my teeth hurt when I drink something cold.

DH: When did you last see a dentist?

PT: I can't remember. I think I had a checkup about 3 years ago.

DH: 病歴について質問します.

PT: 私の病歴についてですね, わかりました. 何でしょうか?

DH: ここに短い質問票があります. 10個の質問です. 質問を読み上げますので,「はい」か「いいえ」に○をつけてもらえますか.

PT: はい.

DH: 最初の質問です. いままでに重病を患ったことがありますか?

PT: 重病ですか. いいえ, 私はずっと健康です.

DH: 入院されたことはありますか?

PT: はい, 一度だけ. スキーで足を骨折しました. 一週間入院しました.

DH: かしこまりました. 高血圧を抱えていますか?

PT: 高血圧ですか? すみませんが, どういうことでしょうか?

DH: 血圧が高いかどうかです. 血圧は高くないですか?

PT: いいえ, 私の血圧は正常です.

DH: 最近, 病院にかかりましたか?

PT: いいえ, ずっと健康です. もう数年病院にはかかっていません.

DH: それは, すばらしいですね. 何かお薬は飲んでいますか?

PT: いいえ.

DH: 薬にアレルギーはありますか?

PT: いいえ, ありません.

DH: 歯科治療後に気分が悪くなったことはありますか?

PT: 気分が悪く, ですか? すみません. どういう意味でしょうか?

DH: えー, 治療の後に意識を失ったりめまいを感じたことはありませんか?

PT: 意識を失ったり, めまいですか. いいえ, そんなことはありません.

DH: かんだときに歯に痛みを感じますか?

PT: はい, 特に右下の奥歯に感じます.

DH: そのことを表に記入しておきます. あとで先生が診察してくれます. 何か温かいものや冷たいもの, 甘いものを飲んだときに痛みを感じますか?

PT: はい, 冷たいものを飲むとときどき歯が痛みます.

DH: 最後に歯科医院にかかったのはいつですか?

PT: 思い出せません. 3年前くらいに検査を受けたと思います.

Listening 3 20

A. Yes, just one time. After an anesthetic, I felt dizzy. It was terrible.

B. I have a cold at the moment, so I'm taking cold medicine.

C. About 2 years ago.

D. Yes, I'm allergic to penicillin.

E. Yes, if I eat ice-cream or drink something very cold, it's very painful.

A. はい, 一度だけです. 麻酔の後に, めまいを感じました. ひどかったです.

B. いま風邪を引いているので，風邪薬を飲んでいます．
C. 2年ほど前です．
D. はい，私はペニシリンにアレルギーがあります．
E. はい，アイスクリームを食べたり冷たいものを飲むと，痛みます．

Target vocabulary 21

1. A-L-L-E-R-G-I-C
2. B-I-T-E
3. D-I-Z-Z-Y
4. F-A-I-N-T
5. H-Y-P-E-R-T-E-N-S-I-O-N
6. I-N G-O-O-D H-E-A-L-T-H
7. M-E-D-I-C-A-L H-I-S-T-O-R-Y
8. P-A-I-N-F-U-L
9. Q-U-E-S-T-I-O-N-N-A-I-R-E

1. アレルギーの
2. かむ
3. めまい
4. 意識を失う
5. 高血圧
6. 体調がよい
7. 病歴
8. 痛い，苦しい
9. 質問表

6 Symptoms:Asking what the problem is Asking how long the patient has had the problem

Listening 1 22

1

DH: What seems to be the problem?
PT: I have toothache. I think it's this tooth at the back.

DH: 何か問題がおありですか？
PT: 歯が痛いのです．この奥歯だと思います．

2

DH: How can I help you?
PT: Well, my gums are bleeding. I'm really worried.

DH: どうしましたか？
PT: えー，歯茎から血が出ています．本当に心配です．

3

DH: Do you have any particular problems?
PT: Yes, it's painful when I chew. Particularly, when I chew hard food.

DH: 何か特別な問題がおありですか？
PT: はい．かむときに痛みます．特に硬いものをかむときです．

4

DH: What's the problem today?
PT: My gums are swollen.

DH: 今日はどうなさいましたか？
PT: 歯茎が腫れています．

5

DH: What can I do for you?
PT: I fell over this morning. My tooth is chipped. It's just a small chip, but I'd like you to take a look at it.

DH: どうかなさいましたか？
PT: 今朝転んでしまい，歯が欠けてしまいました．少し欠けただけなのですが，みていただきたいのです．

Listening 2 23

1

A: So, what is wrong with Mr. Suzuki?
B: He just called to say his crown came off.

A: それで，鈴木さんはどうしたのですか？
B: 電話で「クラウンが外れた」といっていました．

❷

A: Is the next patient Ms. Jones?

B: Yes, that's right. She said her gums are bleeding. It doesn't look too serious, but she's very worried.

A: 次の患者さんはジョーンズさんですか？

B: はい，そうです．歯茎から出血しているそうです．そんなに重度ではなさそうですが，彼女は大変心配しています．

---

❸

A: And little Joe Sikorski. What is his problem?

B: He fell off his bike and chipped his front tooth. It's nothing serious, but his mother is worried. I can fix it easily.

A: それから，ジョー・シコルスキー君ですね．彼はどうしたのですか？

B: 自転車から落ちて，前歯が欠けたそうです．重度ではなさそうですが，彼のお母さんが心配しています．簡単に処置できると思います．

---

❹

A: Okay. I see we have John Nevara at 10:30. What are his symptoms?

B: He said his gums are swollen.

A: それでは，10：30からはジョン・ネバラさんですね．彼の症状は何ですか？

B: 歯茎が腫れているそうです．

---

❺

A: And the last patient is Ms. Tachizawa. What's the problem?

B: She has a loose tooth.

A: 最後の患者さんは立澤さんですね．どんな問題があるのでしょうか？

B: 歯がぐらついているそうです．

Listening 3 24

❶

DH: How long have you had this problem?

PT: For 2 or 3 weeks.

DH: この問題はどのくらい続いていますか？

PT: 2〜3週間です．

---

❷

DH: When did the pain start?

PT: Last Sunday. So, I've had it for 3 days now.

DH: この痛みはいつ始まりましたか？

PT: この前の日曜日からです．なので，3日間くらいになります．

---

❸

DH: How long have your gums been swollen?

PT: Since yesterday morning.

DH: 歯茎はどのくらいの間腫れていますか？

PT: 昨日の朝からです．

---

❹

DH: When did your filling come out?

PT: Last week sometime.

DH: 充填物はいつ取れましたか？

PT: 先週だったと思います．

---

❺

DH: How long has this tooth been loose?

PT: For about 10 days I guess.

DH: この歯はどのくらいの間ぐらついていますか？

PT: 10日間くらいだと思います．

Target vocabulary 25

1. 症状
2. 出血

3. ぐらついた
4. 欠けた
5. 痛み
6. 歯肉（歯茎）
7. 腫れた
8. 咀嚼（かむ）

7　Explaining treatment

Listening　1 26

DH: Okay, Mr. Sikorski. I'd like to tell you about today's treatment. First, I'm going to take some x-rays. We'll need to go into the next room for that. Then, we'll come back in here and I will check inside your mouth. Okay?

PT: Yes, that's fine with me.

DH: Then, I'll examine your teeth and gums.

PT: Okay.

DH: While I'm doing that, I'll note any problems in the chart. The dentist will look at the chart later. By that time, the x-rays will be ready. I'll check the x-rays for decay and calculus.

DH: それでは，シコルスキーさん．今日の治療について説明します．はじめに，エックス線写真を撮ります．そのために隣の部屋へ行きます．それからここへ戻ってきて，口腔内を検査します．よろしいですね？

PT: はい，大丈夫です．

DH: それから歯と歯茎の検査をします．

PT: わかりました．

DH: 何か問題があったらこの表に書き込んでいきます．あとで，この表を先生がみます．そのときまでには，エックス線写真が準備できているでしょう．むし歯と歯石をエックス線写真で確認します．

Listening　2 27

DH: Then, I will start to scale your teeth.

PT: Will it hurt?

DH: No, you won't feel anything. While I'm scaling, I'll be doing two things. First, I'll remove the hard deposits on your teeth. Then, I'll remove plaque below the gumline.

PT: Okay, I've got that. Then what?

DH: I'll floss all your teeth.

PT: Is that the end of the treatment?

DH: No, I also need to polish your teeth.

PT: Polish my teeth. What does that mean?

DH: Well, I'll remove any stains on your teeth and surface plaque.

PT: How long will it take?

DH: About 40 minutes.

DH: それから，歯をスケーリングします．

PT: 痛いですか？

DH: いいえ，何も感じないでしょう．スケーリングでは，2つのことをします．1つは歯についた歯石を取り除くこと，そして，歯頸線の下の歯垢を取り除くことです．

PT: わかりました．それから何かありますか？

DH: デンタルフロスですべての歯を磨きます．

PT: それで治療は終わりですか？

DH: いいえ，その後に歯を研磨します．

PT: 歯の研磨ですか？　どういう意味ですか？

DH: えー，歯についた染みや表面の歯垢を取り除くのです．

PT: どのくらいかかりますか？

DH: およそ40分くらいです．

Listening　3 28

1. take some x-rays
2. check inside your mouth
3. examine your teeth and gums
4. check for decay and calculus
5. scale your teeth
6. remove the hard deposits
7. polish your teeth
8. floss your teeth
9. remove any stains

1. エックス線写真を撮る
2. 口腔内を検査する
3. 歯と歯茎を検査する
4. むし歯と歯石を確認する
5. 歯をスケーリングする
6. 歯石を取り除く

7. 歯を研磨する
8. デンタルフロスで歯を磨く
9. 染みを取り除く

Target vocabulary 29

1. calculus
2. chart
3. decay
4. examine
5. gumline
6. hard deposits
7. plaque
8. polish
9. stains

---

1. 歯石
2. 表
3. 齲蝕（むし歯）
4. 検査する
5. 歯頸線
6. 歯石
7. プラーク（歯垢）
8. 研磨する
9. 染み，着色

Special Listening— 30
Listening to dental topics 2

Today, I'd like to tell you about a special event in England called National Smile Week. It happens once a year. This year a special survey was done.

Here are the results of the survey. I'll start by telling you about 4 main problems that were found. First, 50% of people don't know how to brush properly. Second, 45% of people brush for less than 2 minutes a day. Third, 40% of people never floss. And fourth, 60% of people never clean their tongue.

From the survey, here are 4 things that people must remember to do. One, it is important to floss every day. Two, you should try to reduce the amount of sugary food and drinks. Three,

you should visit the dentist regularly. Four, you should choose healthy snacks like fresh fruit, raw vegetables and cheese.

今日は，英国の特別なイベント，ナショナルスマイルウィークについて話したいと思います．年に一度のものです．今年は特別な調査が行われました．

ここに調査の結果があります．調査の結果からわかった4つの問題点についてお話しします．第一は，50%の人が正しい歯の磨き方を知らないということです．第二に，45%の人が1日に2分間以下しか歯磨きをしないということです．第三に，40%がデンタルフロスを全く使わないということです．そして第四が，60%が全く舌を磨いていないということです．

調査の結果から，人々が覚えておかなければならない4つのことがわかりました．第一に，毎日デンタルフロスを使うことが大切だということ，第二に，糖分を多く含んだ飲食物を減らすように努力すべきだということ，第三は，定期的に歯科医院に通うべきだということ，第四に，間食では新鮮な果物や生野菜，チーズのような健康的なものをとるべきだということです．

---

8 Giving brushing instructions Asking patients questions about brushing

Listening 1 31

1. Put the bristles of the toothbrush along the gumline at a 45 degree angle. The bristles should touch the tooth and the gumline.
2. Brush the outer surface of 2 to 3 teeth. Use a back and forward rolling motion. Then move the brush to the next group of 2 to 3 teeth and do the same thing.
3. Now brush the inner surface of the teeth. Keep the brush at a 45 degree angle. Make sure the brush is in contact with the tooth surface and the gumline.
4. Now brush behind the front teeth, top and bottom.

5. Finally, place the toothbrush against the biting surface of the teeth, and brush back and forth. Also, brush the tongue from back to front to remove bacteria.

---

1. 歯頸線に対して45°くらいの角度で歯ブラシの毛先を当ててください．毛先は歯と歯頸線の両方に当たるようにすべきです．
2. 2〜3本ずつ，歯の外面を磨いてください．前後させながらローリングモーションで行ってください．それから次の2〜3本の歯に歯ブラシを移動させて，同じことをくりかえしてください．
3. それから歯の内面を磨いてください．45°の角度を忘れないでください．歯ブラシの毛先が歯の表面と歯頸線の両方に接触するようにしてください．
4. それから上下前歯の裏側を磨いてください．
5. 最後に，歯ブラシを歯の咬合面におき，前後に動かして磨きます．また，バクテリアを除くため，舌を後ろから前の動きで磨いてください．

Listening 2 32

1. Use a toothbrush with soft, nylon, round-ended bristles.
2. You should replace your toothbrush every 3 or 4 months.
3. You should use toothpaste that contains fluoride.
4. You should try to floss your teeth every day.
5. After you brush use a mouthwash.
6. Keep Xylitol in your bag and use it after you snack.

---

1. やわらかく，ナイロン製で，毛先の丸いブラシを使ってください．
2. 3〜4カ月ごとに歯ブラシを交換すべきです．
3. フッ素配合の歯磨き粉を使うべきです．
4. 毎日デンタルフロスで歯をきれいにすべきです．
5. 歯を磨いた後はマウスウォッシュを使いましょう．
6. バッグの中にいつもキシリトールガムを常備し，おやつの後などに使いましょう．

Listening 3 33

1. How many times do you brush your teeth a day?

---

2. When do you usually brush your teeth?
3. How long do you brush your teeth for?
4. How do you brush your teeth?
5. Do you use a manual or an electric toothbrush?

---

1. 1日に何回歯を磨きますか？
2. ふだんはいつ歯を磨きますか？
3. どのくらい長く歯を磨きますか？
4. どのように歯を磨きますか？
5. 手動と電動のどちらの歯ブラシを使いますか？

Target vocabulary 34

1. bristles （ブラシなどの）毛
2. gumline 歯頸線
3. outer surface 表層，外面
4. inner surface 内面
5. biting surface 咬合面
6. bacteria バクテリア（細菌）
7. back and forth 前後
8. rolling motion ローリングモーション

---

9 Giving advice : Telling patients what they should or should not do

Listening 1 35

1. I've finished scaling and polishing your teeth. I want to give you some advice about how to look after your teeth. First, smoking. You said you smoke a packet of cigarettes a day. You shouldn't smoke. It's bad for your teeth and gums. Have you tried to give up?
2. Next, snacking. You told me that you tend to snack a lot. That means you eat a lot of sugar. You shouldn't snack or have sugary drinks between meals. If you really want to snack, choose something healthy like raw vegetables, cheese, or nuts and raisins.
3. Now brushing. Let me give you some

advice about brushing. You should brush 3 times a day for 2 minutes. And you should floss daily.

4. You should have a checkup every six months. It's very important. We will send you a recall card. So, when you get a recall card, please call to make an appointment.

5. I noticed your teeth were very stained before I polished them. I guess you drink a lot of coffee or tea. You shouldn't drink too much coffee, tea or red wine.

---

1. 歯のスケーリングと研磨が終わりました. 歯のケアの仕方について少しアドバイスをしたいと思います. まず, 喫煙についてです. 1日に1箱お吸いになるとおっしゃっていましたが, 喫煙はすべきではありません. 歯にも歯茎にもよくありません. やめようと思ったことはありますか?

2. 次に, 間食についてです. よく間食されるというお話でしたが, ということはたくさん糖分を摂取しているということです. 食事の間に間食や糖分を含んだ飲料は取るべきではありません. もし間食したくなったら, 生野菜やチーズ, ナッツ類やレーズンなどを選んでください.

3. さて, 歯磨きについてです. 歯磨きについても助言があります. 1日3回, 2分ほど磨いてください. それから毎日デンタルフロスを使うべきです.

4. 検診は半年ごとに受けるようにしてください. とても重要なことです. 定期検診のハガキを送りますので, 受け取ったら, 予約の電話をください.

5. 研磨する前のあなたの歯は, 染みがひどく着いているのがわかりました. コーヒーや紅茶を多く飲まれるのでしょう. コーヒー, 紅茶, 赤ワインはあまり飲まないほうがよいでしょう.

Listening 2 36

1. The best way to protect your teeth is by effective brushing and flossing.

2. Okay. This is important advice. Don't forget to change your toothbrush every few months. An old toothbrush is no good. It doesn't clean properly.

3. Another important point is snacking. It's important to reduce the amount of sugar you eat. So, don't snack. It's bad for your

teeth.

4. You should visit the dentist regularly. So, don't forget to come in for a checkup every six months.

5. Try to use a mouthwash. It will help to keep your breath fresh and reduce plaque.

6. It's a good idea to carry a packet of Xylitol in your bag.

7. Toothpaste that contains fluoride helps fight tooth decay.

---

1. 歯を守る一番の方法は正しく歯を磨くこととデンタルフロスを使うことです.

2. では, 重要なアドバイスです. 数カ月ごとに歯ブラシを交換することを忘れないでください. 古い歯ブラシはよくありません. 正しく磨くことができないのです.

3. もう一つの重要な点は間食についてです. 糖分の摂取を減らすことが大切です. ですから, 間食はやめましょう. 歯によくありません.

4. 定期的に歯科医院に通いましょう. 半年ごとの検診を忘れないようにしましょう.

5. マウスウォッシュを使うようにしましょう. 息をさわやかにし, 歯垢も減らしてくれます.

6. バッグの中にキシリトールガムを常備するのもよいでしょう.

7. フッ素配合の歯磨き粉はむし歯予防になります.

Listening 3 37

1. You shouldn't smoke.

2. You shouldn't snack or have sugary drinks.

3. You should brush 3 times a day for 2 minutes.

4. You should have a checkup every six months.

5. You shouldn't drink too much coffee, tea or red wine.

---

1. 喫煙はすべきではありません.

2. 間食や糖分を含んだ飲料はとるべきではありません.

3. 1日3回, 2分間ずつ歯を磨くべきです.

4. 半年に一度は検診を受けるべきです.

5. コーヒー, 紅茶, 赤ワインはあまり飲まないほうがいいでしょう.

A. You should floss every day.
B. I'm going to give you some advice.
C. You can protect your teeth by brushing.
D. It is important to have a checkup every six months.
E. Please change your toothbrush every 3 or 4 months.
F. Sugar is bad for your teeth. Please cut down on sugar.
G. I'm going to polish your teeth.

A. 毎日デンタルフロスを使うべきです.
B. いくつかアドバイスをいたします.
C. 歯を磨くことで歯を守ることができます.
D. 半年ごとに検診を受けるのは大切なことです.
E. 3～4カ月ごとに歯ブラシを交換してください.
F. 糖分は歯に悪いものです. 糖分を控えましょう.
G. あなたの歯を研磨します.

10 Understanding patient questions How to ask questions

Listening 1 39

1

DH: Okay, that's the end of the treatment. Do you have any questions?
PT: I have a question about tooth decay. What causes tooth decay?

DH: それでは, これで治療は終了です. 何か質問はございますか?
PT: むし歯について1つ質問があります. むし歯の原因は何ですか?

2

DH: I've given you advice on how to look after your teeth. What questions do you have?
PT: You told me I had some plaque on my teeth. I don't know what plaque is. Could you explain it, please? What causes plaque?

DH: 歯のケアの仕方についてアドバイスをいたしました. 何か質問はございますか?
PT: 歯に歯垢がついているとのことですが, 歯垢とはどんなものかがわかりません. 説明していただけますか? 何が原因で歯垢ができるのでしょうか?

3

DH: Okay, so that's all I have to say about oral hygiene. Would you like to ask any questions?
PT: Dr. Watanabe said I have some inflammation. What is inflammation?

DH: では口腔衛生についてはのお話は以上です. 何か質問はございますか?
PT: 渡辺先生がおっしゃるには私には炎症があるとのことですが, 炎症とはどんなものですか?

4

DH: Is there anything you'd like to know?
PT: Sometimes this tooth hurts. It's very sensitive. Could you explain why it is sensitive?

DH: 何かお知りになりたいことはございますか?
PT: ときどき, この歯が痛みます. とても敏感な状態です. どうしてなのか教えてくれませんか?

5

DH: Do you need any more information?
PT: You said I have a lot of stains on my teeth. I think my teeth look too dark. I really want whiter teeth. How can I get whiter teeth?

DH: 何かお知りになりたいことはございますか?
PT: 歯にたくさん染みが着いているとのことですが, 私の歯は暗すぎると思います. もっと白い歯にしたいのですが, どうしたら白くなりますか?

Listening 2 40

1. Do you have any questions?
2. What questions do you have?
3. Would you like to ask any questions?
4. Is there anything you would like to know?
5. Do you need any more information?

1. 何か質問はございますか？
2. どんな質問がございますか？
3. 何かお聞ききになりたい質問はございますか？
4. 何かお知りになりたいことはございますか？
5. 何かほかに情報が必要ですか？

Listening 3 41

1. Do I need any medicine?
2. When can I eat or drink?
3. Is that the end of today's treatment?
4. When do I have to come back?
5. Where do I pay?
6. When is my next checkup?

1. 私には何か薬が必要ですか？
2. いつ食べたり飲んだりできますか？
3. これで今日の治療は終わりですか？
4. いつ来ればよいですか？
5. どこで支払うのですか？
6. 次の検診はいつですか？

Target vocabulary 42

1. tooth decay
2. plaque
3. inflammation
4. gum disease
5. stains
6. whiter teeth
7. fluoride

1. 齲蝕（むし歯）
2. プラーク（歯垢）
3. 炎症
4. 歯周病
5. 染み，着色
6. より白い歯

7. フッ素

11 Giving advice to a patient who is going to have a tooth extracted

Listening 1 43

PT: Dr. Watanabe said I need to have a tooth out. I'm really worried. Will it hurt? Will it bleed?

DH: Okay, Mr. Smith, you are having some orthodontic work. Dr. Watanabe will need to extract a tooth. You really don't need to worry at all. After extraction, you will probably experience some pain and discomfort. So, I'd like to give you some general advice.

PT: Okay. Thanks.

DH: First of all, you should avoid hot or spicy food and drinks. Also, avoid smoking and alcohol.

PT: Just a moment. Can you say that again? Avoid what?

DH: Hot or spicy food and drinks.

PT: Okay. I've got that.

DH: Another thing. If your gum starts to bleed, bite firmly on a sterile gauze pad. You should change the pad every 20 minutes or so. If the bleeding doesn't stop, please contact us. You can call us anytime on 0325048037

PT: Okay.

DH: On the day after the operation, rinse your mouth with hot, salt water or an antiseptic mouthwash.

PT: Hot, salt water. Right. I've got that.

DH: And don't forget you need to come back a week later.

PT: A week later. Right. Can I make an appointment now?

DH: Yes, that's a good idea. Let's go through

to the reception. Don't worry. It will be okay.

PT: 渡辺先生がおっしゃるには, 私は歯を抜かないといけないらしいです. すごく怖いのですが, 痛いのでしょうか? 血が出るのでしょうか?

DH: スミスさん, あなたは歯科矯正治療をするのです. 渡辺先生が歯を抜くことになるでしょう. でも, 全然心配する必要はありません. 抜歯後はいくらか痛みや不快感があるかもしれませんが, いくつかアドバイスをしたいと思います.

PT: わかりました. ありがとうございます.

DH: まずはじめに, 熱いものや香辛料の効いた飲食物は避けましょう. また喫煙や飲酒も控えましょう.

PT: ちょっと待ってください. もう一度いってください. 何を控えるのですか?

DH: 熱いものや香辛料の効いた飲食物です.

PT: わかりました.

DH: もう一つ, 歯茎から血が出るようでしたら, 滅菌したガーゼの傷あてを強くかんでください. 傷あては20分ごとに交換しましょう. それでも出血が止らないようでしたら, いつでも連絡をしてください. 電話番号は, 03-2504-8037 です.

PT: わかりました.

DH: 手術が終わった日は, 温かい塩水か, マウスウォッシュで口をゆすいでください.

PT: 温かい塩水ですね. わかりました.

DH: それから1週間後に来院することを忘れないように.

PT: 1週間後ですね. わかりました. いま予約を入れてもいいですか?

DH: そうですね. 受付へ参りましょう. 心配しないで. 大丈夫ですよ.

Listening 2 44

1. Dr. Watanabe will need to extract a tooth.
2. You will probably experience some pain.
3. I'd like to give you some general advice.
4. Also, avoid smoking and alcohol.
5. You should change the pad every 20 minutes.

---

1. 渡辺先生が歯を抜くことになるでしょう.
2. すこし痛みを感じるかもしれません.
3. 一般的なアドバイスをいっておきます.
4. それから喫煙や飲酒は避けましょう.

5. 傷あては20分ごとに交換しましょう.

Listening 3 45

1. teeth
2. drink
3. pads
4. appointment
5. extraction

---

1. 歯
2. 飲料
3. 傷あて
4. 予約
5. 抜歯

Target vocabulary 46

A. On the day after the operation, rinse your mouth with hot, salt water.
B. You are having orthodontic treatment.
C. You should avoid hot or spicy food and drinks.
D. Dr. Watanabe will need to extract a tooth.
E. You will probably experience some pain.
F. Bite firmly on a sterile gauze pad.
G. Let me know if you experience any discomfort.

A. 手術が終わった日は, 温かい塩水で口をゆすいでください.
B. あなたは歯科矯正治療をするのです.
C. 熱いものや香辛料の効いた飲食物は避けましょう.
D. 渡辺先生が歯を抜くことになるでしょう.
E. すこし痛みを感じるかもしれません.
F. 滅菌したガーゼの傷あてを強くかんでください.
G. 何か不快に感じるようでしたら, 教えてください.

12 Telling a patient about medicine Giving directions to a pharmacy

Listening 1 47

DH: How are you feeling, Mr. Smith?

PT: Okay, I guess. It wasn't so painful.

DH: That's good. Now, I need to tell you about your medicine.

PT: Do I need medicine?

DH: Yes, the dentist said after an extraction you should have antibiotics and painkillers.

PT: Antibiotics and painkillers? Two kinds of medicine? Do I really need them?

DH: Yes, after an extraction, it's important. Just a minute and I'll explain about them.

PT: Okay.

DH: First, antibiotics. These will prevent infection.

PT: Prevent infection. Okay, I've got that.

DH: Take one tablet 3 times a day for 3 days. Take the tablet after meals.

PT: Okay. 1 tablet, 3 times a day for 3 days after meals.

DH: One more thing. It is very important to finish all the tablets.

PT: Okay. I've got that. I must finish all the tablets.

DH: Now about the painkillers. It is important to start taking the painkillers before the anesthetic wears off.

PT: Why is that?

DH: It works better like that. So, you should take a painkiller as soon as you get home.

PT: How many tablets should I take?

DH: You can take a maximum of 3 tablets a day. Take them 4 hours apart. And remember to start taking the painkillers before the anesthetic wears off.

DH: ご気分はいかがですか？ スミスさん.

PT: 大丈夫だと思います. そんなに痛くありませんでした.

DH: それはよかったです. それでは，薬についてご説明します.

PT: 薬を飲むのですか？

DH: はい，先生がおっしゃるには，抗生物質と鎮痛薬が必要だそうです.

PT: 抗生物質と鎮痛剤ですか？ ２種類の薬ですか？ そんなに必要なのですか？

DH: はい，抜歯後には欠かせません. 少々，説明しますね.

PT: わかりました.

DH: まず抗生物質からです. これは感染を防ぐものです.

PT: 感染を防ぐのですね. わかりました.

DH: １日３回１錠ずつを３日間，食後に摂取してください.

PT: わかりました. １錠ずつを１日３回３日間，食事の後でですね.

DH: もう１つ大切なのは，すべての薬を飲み終わらせることです.

PT: わかりました. 薬は全部飲まなければいけないのですね.

DH: 次に鎮痛剤です. これは麻酔がきれる前に飲み始めることが大切です.

PT: それはなぜですか？

DH: そのほうが効果的なのです. ですから，家に帰ったらすぐに鎮痛剤を１錠飲んでください.

PT: どれくらい飲めばよいのでしょうか？

DH: １日３回まで飲むことができます. ４時間ごとに飲んでください. 麻酔が切れる前に鎮痛剤を飲み始めるということは忘れないでくださいね.

Listening 2 48

1. Please take 1 tablet, twice a day for 3 days. Take the tablets after breakfast and after dinner. Okay?

2. You need to take 2 of these tablets, 3 times a day for 4 days. Take them after meals.

3. This is simple. Take 1 tablet once a day for 5 days. Take it every morning after breakfast.

4. Take 1 tablet 3 times a day for 3 days. Take the tablet after meals.

---

1. １日２回１錠ずつで３日間飲んでください. 朝食と夕食の後に飲んでください. よろしいですね？

2. １日３回２錠ずつで４日間飲んでください. 食後に飲んでくださいね.

3. はい，これは簡単です．1日1錠で5日間飲んでください．毎朝，朝食後に飲んでくださいね．
4. 1日3回1錠ずつで3日間飲んでください．食後に飲んでくださいね．

Listening 3 49

❶

PT: Excuse me, where is the nearest pharmacy?

DH: We have a small one in this building. Go to the main entrance. You'll see 4 windows. It's the one on the right, next to the cashier.

PT: On the right. Next to the cashier. Got it. Thanks.

PT: すみません．一番近い薬局はどこでしょうか？

DH: この建物のなかに小さい薬局が1つあります．正面玄関に行ってください．4つの窓口がありますので，会計の右隣の窓口に行ってください．

PT: 会計の右隣ですね．わかりました．ありがとうございます．

❷

PT: Where can I find the pharmacy?

DH: Take the elevator down to the first floor. As you come out of the elevator, you'll see the reception desk in front of you. Turn right and the pharmacy is on your right in front of the office.

PT: 薬局はどこにありますか？

DH: エレベータで1階まで降りてください．エレベータから降りると，目の前に受付が見えます．右に行くと，右側に薬局があります．オフィスの前です．

❸

DH: I'm afraid we don't have a pharmacy here in the clinic. But there is a pharmacy about 2 or 3 minutes from here on foot. You can get your medicine there.

PT: Okay, thanks. How do I get there?

DH: It's easy. Go out of the dental clinic and turn right. Go straight for 2 blocks. You will see a hamburger shop on the corner. Turn right, there's a pharmacy on the right next to the hamburger shop.

DH: 申し訳ございませんが，当医院には薬局がございません．ですが，ここから歩いて2〜3分のところに1つ薬局がございます．そこで薬をお買い求めいただけます．

PT: わかりました．ありがとうございます．そちらへはどうやって行けばよろしいですか？

DH: 簡単です．この歯科医院を出て，右に曲がってください．道路を2つ渡りますと，角にハンバーガーショップが見えます．そこを右に曲がっていただくと，右側に薬局がございます．ハンバーガーショップのすぐ隣です．

Target vocabulary 50

A. 薬
B. 1日3回
C. 抗生物質
D. (薬が) きれる
E. 痛み止め，鎮痛剤
F. 1日2回
G. 麻酔
H. 感染

---

13 Explaining where to pay, the cost of treatment and the price of dental products

Listening 1 51

❶

PT: Excuse me, where do I pay?

DH: Please go back to the waiting area. You can pay at the reception. The receptionist will call your name.

PT: Thank you.

PT：すみません．どこでお支払いすればよいですか？
DH：待合室へ戻ってください．受付でお支払いいただけ
　　ます．受付の者があなたのお名前をよぶと思います．
PT：ありがとうございます．

---

❷

PT：Excuse me. I'm not sure where to pay.
DH：Okay, this is the third floor. Go down to the
　　first floor. You can pay there.
PT：The first floor. Okay, I've got that.

PT：すみません．どこでお支払いすればよいのかがわか
　　りません．
DH：はい．ここは３階ですので１階に下りてください．
　　そこでお支払いいただけます．
PT：１階ですね．わかりました．

---

❸

DH：That is the end of the treatment. Please
　　go back to the waiting area, you can pay
　　at the window on the left. Please wait until
　　they call your name.
PT：Okay, thanks.

DH：これで治療は終了です．待合室にお戻りください．
　　左側の窓口でお支払いください．あなたのお名前が
　　よばれるまでお待ちください．
PT：わかりました．ありがとうございます．

---

❹

PT：Excuse me. Where do I pay?
DH：Okay. Please go back to the first floor. Pay
　　at the window that says '*kaikei*'.
PT：Sorry, I don't understand Japanese. Which
　　window do I need to go to?
DH：Okay. It's the window in the middle. It says
　　kaikei. It's Japanese for cashier.
PT：The window in the middle. Okay, I've got
　　that. Thanks.

PT：すみません．どこでお支払いすればよいのですか．
DH：はい．１階にお戻りください．「会計」と書かれた窓
　　口でお支払いいただけます．

PT：すみません．日本語がわからないのですが，どの窓
　　口へ行けばよいのですか？
DH：真ん中の窓口です．「会計」とあります．日本語で「会
　　計」の意味です．
PT：真ん中の窓口ですね．わかりました．ありがとうご
　　ざいます．

---

❺

PT：Excuse me. I'm not sure where to pay.
DH：It's easy. You can pay next to the
　　reception.
PT：Next to the reception. Okay, I've got that.
　　Thanks.

PT：すみません．どこでお支払いすればよいのかがわか
　　らないのですが．
DH：ご心配いりません．受付の横でお支払いいただけま
　　す．
PT：受付の横ですね．わかりました．ありがとうござい
　　ます．

Listening 2 52

1. The cost of today's treatment is ¥5,850.
2. That's ¥1,150, please.
3. So, the cost of your crown is ¥15,500.
4. So, today you just had a checkup. That's
   ¥678.
5. The cost of your orthodontic treatment this
   time is ¥31, 975.

---

1. 今日の治療費は 5,850 円です．
2. 1,150 円です．
3. クラウンの金額が 15,500 円です．
4. では今日は検診だけでしたね．678 円です．
5. 今回の矯正治療の費用は，31,975 円です．

Listening 3 53

DH：That covers brushing and flossing.
PT：Okay, thanks.
DH：The last thing I want to tell you about is
　　dental hygiene products. We have a small
　　shop selling dental hygiene products on
　　the first floor. I have a few products that I

would like to recommend. First of all, you need to have some dental floss.

PT: Dental floss. How much does that cost?

DH: It costs ¥418 for 1 pack. Why not buy a couple of packs? One for your home, and one for your office. Another thing I want to recommend is an interdental brush. It's useful for brushing between your teeth. It costs ¥378 for 15 brushes.

PT: Okay, I'll get a pack of interdental brushes. Should I get anything else?

DH: Well, as I told you, you need to change your toothbrush frequently. We have some good brushes in our shop. They cost ¥295 each. It's good value. Why don't you buy 3 or 4?

PT: Okay. That's a good idea.

DH: And one more thing you need is a tube of fluoride toothpaste. Why don't you buy 2 or 3 tubes? One tube costs ¥313.

PT: Okay.

DH: Finally, why don't you buy some mouthwash? A bottle of mint mouthwash costs ¥733 for 1 liter.

PT: Okay, I'll do that. Thanks for your advice.

DH: You're welcome. See you in 6 months.

DH: これで，歯磨きとデンタルフロスの説明は終わりです．

PT: はい，ありがとうございます．

DH: 最後に歯科衛生用の製品についてご説明します．1 階にある小さなお店で歯科衛生用の製品を売っています．いくつかおすすめしたい製品があるのですが，まず，あなたにはデンタルフロスが必要です．

PT: デンタルフロスですね．いくらですか？

DH: 1パック418円です．何パックか買われてはいかがでしょうか？ 家に1つと職場に1つがよいでしょう．もう1つおすすめしたいのは，歯間ブラシです．歯の間を磨くのに便利です．15個で378円です．

PT: わかりました．歯間ブラシを1パック買います．ほかに買ったほうがよいものはありますか？

DH: えー，さっきも申し上げましたように，歯ブラシの交換も頻繁に行う必要があります．私どもの店にはよい歯ブラシを295円で販売しております．お買い得ですので，3～4本ほど買われてはいかがでしょ

うか？

PT: わかりました．それはよいですね．

DH: それからもう1つあなたに必要なのは，フッ素の配合された歯磨き粉でしょう．これも2～3本買われてはいかがでしょうか？ 1つ313円です．

PT: わかりました．

DH: 最後に，マウスウォッシュもお薦めします．ミント味のものは1瓶1リットルで733円です．

PT: わかりました．買ってみます．教えていただきありがとうございます．

DH: どういたしまして．6カ月後にまたお会いしましょう．

---

1. pay
2. receptionist
3. treatment
4. dental hygiene products
5. reception

---

1. 支払う
2. 会計係
3. 治療
4. 歯科衛生用の製品
5. 会計

14 What do dental hygienists need for the job? What's a typical day for a DH?

Int: I'd like to ask about your job.

DH: Sure. What would you like to know?

Int: How long have you been a dental hygienist?

DH: For 20 years.

Int: I see. And what is the most important part of your job?

DH: I think the most important thing is teaching people how to brush and floss. In other words, educating people to look after their teeth.

Int : あなたの仕事についてお尋ねします.
DH : はい, 何でしょうか?
Int : 歯科衛生士になってどれくらいになりますか?
DH : 20 年です.
Int : そうですか. では, 歯科衛生士の仕事で一番大切なことは何ですか?
DH : 一番大切なことは正しい歯磨きとデンタルフロスの使い方を教えることだと思います. つまり, 歯のケアの仕方を教育することですね.

Listening 2 56

Int : I see. So, teaching people how to brush and floss properly is important.
DH : That's right.
Int : What do dental hygienists need for the job?
DH : I think there are 4 main things. First, you need to be interested in science. Second, you need to be able to communicate well with patients.
Int : Okay. So, you need to be interested in science and be able to communicate well. I've got that. What are the other two things?
DH : Well, you have to be patient. I mean you have to explain things clearly and simply to patients. It's no good getting angry.
Int : And the fourth thing?
DH : You use your hands a lot. So, of course, you need to be good with your hands.

Int : なるほど. 正しい歯磨きとデンタルフロスの使い方を教えることが重要なのですね?
DH : そうです.
Int : では, 歯科衛生士として働くには何が必要だと思いますか?
DH : それは 4 つあると思います. まず, 科学に興味をもつことです. 第二に, 患者さんとうまく意思疎通をはかることができることです.
Int : なるほど. 科学に興味をもつことと, コミュニケーションをうまく取る必要があるのですね. わかりました. ほかの 2 つは何ですか?

DH : えー, 辛抱強くなくてはなりません. つまり患者さんにはっきりと簡潔に説明する必要があります. 腹を立てるのはよくありません.
Int : 4 番目は何でしょうか?
DH : 手をよく使いますので, もちろん, 手先が器用である必要があります.

Listening 3 57

Int : Could you describe a typical day for a DH?
DH : A typical day, okay. If I have a new patient, I start with an intra-oral and extra-oral examination.
Int : What does that mean?
DH : It means I check inside the mouth and also outside. That's just to make sure everything is okay.
Int : Okay. I see.
DH : Then I examine the patient's teeth and gums. I write this information on the chart for the dentist to see later.
Int : Okay, what's next?
DH : I take x-rays and check for tooth decay and calculus.
Int : What's calculus?
DH : It's plaque that has become very hard.
Int : Okay. I see.
DH : Then, I scale the patient's teeth to remove any calculus on the teeth. I also remove plaque that is below the gumline. Then I polish the teeth to remove stains and surface plaque.
Int : How long does that take?
DH : Including setting up the room before the patient comes and cleaning it later, about 30 to 45 minutes.

Int : 歯科衛生士としての典型的な一日を教えてください.
DH : 典型的な一日ですね, わかりました. 新しい患者さんがいらしたときは, 口腔内と口腔外の検査からはじめます.
Int : それはどういう意味ですか?
DH : 口の中と外を検査するのです. 何か問題がないかを確認するためです.
Int : なるほど, わかりました.

DH: それから患者さんの歯と歯茎をみます。あとで先生がみれるように，その結果を表に書き込みます。

Int: わかりました。その次は何ですか？

DH: エックス線写真を撮り，むし歯と歯石の状況をみます。

Int: 歯石とは何ですか？

DH: 硬化した歯垢のことです。

Int: なるほど。

DH: それから歯についた歯石を取り除くためにスケーリングをします。歯頸線の下の歯垢も取り除きます。それから，歯の染みや表面の歯垢を取り除くために研磨します。

Int: どれくらいの時間がかかるのですか？

DH: 患者さんが来る前の診察室の準備と，後の清掃を含めるとおよそ 30 ～ 45 分くらいです。

Target vocabulary **58**

A. 歯石

B. 表

C. 齲蝕（むし歯）

D. 口腔外

E. 手先が器用

F. 口腔内

G. 研磨する

H. プラーク（歯垢）を取り除く

I. 歯石を除去する

J. 診察室の準備をする

Answers

1. Have you visited us before?

Listening 1

1. New Patient, 2. New Patient, 3. Registered Patient, 4. Registered Patient, 5. Registered Patient

Listening 2

1. Have, you, visited (C), 2. Could, I, have (B), 3. Could, you, spell (A), 4. When, can, you (E), 5. How, about, Tuesday (D), 6. Do, you, have (F)

Listening 3

1. (S) recall card, 2. (S) clinic, 3. (P) details, 4. (S) dentist, 5. (S) appointment, 6. (P) teeth

Target vocabulary

(4) appointment, (6) details, (1) register, (2) toothache, (7) recall card, (5) teeth, (3) cleaned

2. Taking a patient's name, address, telephone number   Filling out a registration card

Listening 1

1. Hughes, 2. Cowley, 3. Davies, 4. Boyd, 5. Jones

Listening 2

1. Nevara, 2. Williams, 3. Sikorski, 4. Waldhoff, 5. Wright

Listening 3

Name : (John) Richards, Sex : male, Age : 38, Address : (Minato City, Higashi) 3-5-207, Telephone No : (080-340) 1-8783

Target vocabulary

1. fill out, 2. registration card, 3. family name, 4. name, 5. telephone number, 6. address

3. Making appointments: Days,dates,times

Listening 1

1. Tuesday, 9am, 2. Wednesday, 4/10, 3. 12/18, 4:30, 4. 6/17, 7:30, 5. Friday, 2pm

Listening 2

1. May 30th, 2. June 15th, 3. May 6th, 4. October 19th, 5. December 14th

Listening 3

1. 3:15, 2. 8:00, 3. 9:15, 4. 8:45, 5. 2:20

Target vocabulary

(6) braces, (8) dental hygienist, (7) brush properly, (4) orthodontic treatment, (3) molars,
(1) crown, (5) oral hygiene, (2) restoration

Special Listening —Listening to dental topics 1

1. ① 5, ② 30, 12
2. ① 1, twice, ② once, ③ 39

4. Types of treatment

Listening 1

(3) orthodontic treatment, (5) whitening treatment, (4) partial denture, (2) restoration,
(1) cleaning & polishing, (6) permanent filling, (7) extraction

Listening 2

1. cleaning, polishing, 2. restoration, work, 3. partial, denture, 4. orthodontic, treatment,
5. whitening, treatment, 6. permanent, filling, 7. extraction

Listening 3

1. D, 2. A, 3. B, 4. E, 5. C

Target vocabulary

1. f, 2. c, 3. a, 4. b, 5. e, 6. d

5. Questions about medical history

Listening 1

(2) illnesses, (6) hospitalized, (8) suffering from, (4) medications, (5) painful, (1) hypertension,
(7) dental treatment, (3) sore, (9) penicillin, (10) allergic

Listening 2

1. No, 2. Yes, 3. No, 4. No, 5. No, 6. No, 7. No, 8. Yes, 9. Yes, 10. 3 (years ago)

Listening 3

1. B, 2. D, 3. A, 4. E, 5. C

Target vocabulary

1. allergic, 2. bite, 3. dizzy, 4. faint, 5. hypertension, 6. in good health, 7. medical history, 8. painful, 9. questionnaire

6. Symptoms: Asking what the problem is Asking how long the patient has had the problem

Listening 1

1. have toothache, 2. gums are bleeding, 3. painful when I chew, 4. gums are swollen, 5. tooth is chipped

Listening 2

1. f, 2. c, 3. e, 4. d, 5. b

Listening 3

1. f, 2. i, 3. a, 4. c, 5. e

Target vocabulary

(2) bleeding, (8) chew, (4) chipped, (6) gums, (3) loose, (5) pain, (7) swollen, (1) symptom

7. Explaining treatment

Listening 1

Examine your teeth and gums (3), Note any problems in the chart (4), Take some x-rays (1), Check inside your mouth (2), Check the x-rays for decay and calculus (5)

Listening 2

Remove hard deposits on your teeth (7), Scale your teeth (6), Remove plaque below the gumline (8), Polish your teeth (10), Floss your teeth (9)

Listening 3

1. take, 2. check, 3. examine, 4. check, 5. scale, 6. remove, 7. polish, 8. floss, 9. remove

Target vocabulary

(5) gumline, (6) hard deposits, (2) chart, (4) examine, (7) plaque, (9) stains, (1) calculus, (8) polish, (3) decay,

Special Listening —Listening to dental topics 2

① 50, ② 45, ③ 40, ④ 60
① floss, ② reduce, ③ visit, ④ choose

8.. Giving brushing instructions
Asking patients questions about brushing

Listening 1

(図左から) 2, 4, 5, 3, 1

Listening 2

1. b, 2. d, 3. f, 4. e, 5. c, 6. a

Listening 3

1. How, many, times, 2. When, do, usually, 3. long, do, you, 4. How, do, you, 5. Do, use, manual

Target vocabulary

1. h, 2. a, 3. c, 4. g, 5. e, 6. d, 7. b, 8. f

9. Giving advice: Telling patients what they should or should not do

Listening 1

1. shouldn't, smoking, 2. shouldn't, snacking, 3. should, brushing 3 times a day, 4. should, having a checkup, 5. shouldn't, drinking too much coffee

Listening 2

1. a, f, 2. n, 3. h, 4. e, 5. l, 6. m, 7. b, d

Listening 3

1. smoke, 2. have, sugary, drinks, 3. for, 2, minutes, 4. have, a, checkup, 5. coffee, tea, red, wine

Target vocabulary

A. 6, B. 1, C. 2, D. 5, E. 3, F. 4, G. 7,

10. Understanding patient questions
How to ask questions

Listening 1

1. g, 2. f, 3. c, 4. l, 5. d

Listening 2

1. have, any, questions, 2. What, questions, do, 3. ask, any, questions, 4. like, to, know, 5. Do, you, need

Listening 3

1. c, 2. a, 3. d, 4. b, 5. e, 6. f

Target vocabulary

1. f, 2. a, 3. b, 4. d, 5. c, 6. g, 7. e,

11. Giving advice to a patient who is going to have a tooth extracted

Listening 1

1. b, 2. g, 3. c, 4. e, 5. d

Listening 2

1. a tooth, 2. pain, 3. advice, 4. alcohol, 5. 20

Listening 3

1. teeth, 2. drink, 3. pads, 4. appointment, 5. extraction

Target vocabulary

A. 7, B. 1, C. 5, D. 2, E. 3, F. 6, G. 4

12 Telling a patient about medicine Giving directions to a pharmacy

Listening 1

1. 2, 2. infection, 3. 1, 3, 3, 4. before, 5. 3

Listening 2

1. 1, 2, 3, after breakfast & dinner, 2. 2, 3, 4, after meals, 3. 1, 1, 5, after breakfast, 4. 1, 3, 3, after meals

Listening 3

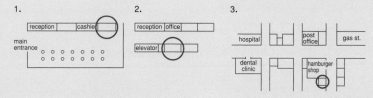

Target vocabulary

A. 8, 薬, B. 7, 1日3回, C. 1, 抗生物質, D. 5, 薬がきれる, E. 2, 痛み止め, 鎮痛剤, F. 6, 1日2回, G. 4, 麻酔, H. 3, 感染

13. Explaining where to pay, the cost of treatment and the price of dental products

Listening 1

1. a, 2. b, 3. e, 4. g, 5. f

Listening 2

1. i, 2. h, 3. c, 4. f, 5. j

Listening 3

2 – d, 4 – j, 6 – f, 8 – g, 9 – c

Target vocabulary

(5) reception, (2) receptionist, (1) pay, (3) treatment, (4) dental hygiene products

14. What do dental hygienists need for the job? What's a typical day for a DH?

Listening 1

1. 20, 2. brush, floss

Listening 2

1. b, 2. d, 3. e, 4. f (順不同)

Listening 3

1. teeth, gums, 2. on the chart, 3. take x-rays, 4. scale, 5. calculus, 6. plaque, gumline, 7. polish, stains, surface plaque

Target vocabulary

A. 4　歯石, B. 9　表, C. 5　齲蝕（むし歯）, D. 3　口腔外, E. 1　手先が器用, F. 2　口腔内, G. 7　研磨する, H. 8　プラーク（歯垢）を取り除く, I. 10　歯石を除去する, J. 6　診療室の準備をする,

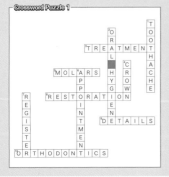

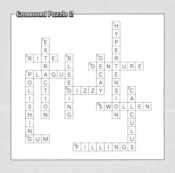

※本書は 2008 年 4 月に「2 週間で英語耳 歯科衛生士のための Listening Skills 音声 CD 付」として発行されたものを, 内容は発行時のまま, 音声データを CD ではなく, 小社 WEB サイトを通じて提供する形式に変更したうえで, 再発行したものです.

2 週間で英語耳
歯科衛生士のための Listening Skills
音声 DL 付   ISBN978-4-263-42327-1

2024 年 5 月 20 日　第 1 版第 1 刷発行

著　者　C. S. Langham
田　嶋　倫　雄
発行者　白　石　泰　夫

発行所　医歯薬出版株式会社

〒113-8612　東京都文京区本駒込1−7−10
TEL. (03)5395−7638(編集)・7630(販売)
FAX. (03)5395−7639(編集)・7633(販売)
https://www.ishiyaku.co.jp/
郵便振替番号 00190−5−13816

乱丁, 落丁の際はお取り替えいたします　　　印刷・あづま堂印刷／製本・愛千製本所